Your Puppy's First Year

Shawn Messonnier, D.V.M.

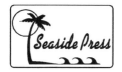

Seaside Press

Library of Congress Cataloging-in-Publication Data

Messonnier, Shawn.
    Your puppy's first year / Shawn Messonnier.
        p.   cm.
    Includes index.
    ISBN 1-55622-386-2
    1. Puppies.   2. Puppies--Health.   I. Title.
    SF427.M488   1995
    636.7'07--dc20   94-48892
                                            CIP

Seaside Press is an imprint of Wordware Publishing, Inc.
No part of this book may be reproduced in any form or by any means
without permission in writing from Wordware Publishing, Inc.

Printed in the United States of America

ISBN 1-55622-386-2
10 9 8 7 6 5 4 3 2 1
9503

All inquiries for volume purchases of this book should be addressed to
Wordware Publishing, Inc., at 1506 Capital Avenue, Plano, Texas 75074.
Telephone inquiries may be made by calling:

(214) 423-0090

Contents

Acknowledgments

A special thanks to the people at Jerry's Perfect Pets (Plano, Texas) and my wonderful clients for their assistance with providing friendly puppies for photography. Thanks also to the folks at the Living Materials Center in Plano for their help with my last book, *Exotic Pets: A Veterinary Guide for Owners*. To the folks at Wordware Publishing, Inc., thanks for your faith in the message *Your Puppy's First Year* has to offer new puppy owners. Thanks always to my wife Sandy and daughter Erica for understanding my inattentiveness during deadlines. Your support means a lot.

Introduction

As a veterinarian, I am always thrilled when a pet owner brings in a puppy for its first visit. These owners are excited about their new pets, and it's exciting for me because I get to teach them how to properly care for their new family members.

Raising a puppy can be fun, but at times it can also be challenging and frustrating. Sometimes owners, armed with incorrect information, have a difficult time raising the new puppy. Most don't have any idea what to expect from their new pet.

I believe that veterinarians should take time on the first visit or even before the first visit to properly discuss with the new or prospective owner exactly what to expect that important first year! A new puppy requires time, commitment, a lot of love and attention, and often a sizable financial investment.

No one should own a puppy without being fully prepared for this awesome responsibility. To help better prepare you for the trials and tribulations of puppy-hood, I wrote *Your Puppy's First Year*. Unlike some puppy books, this book is written by a practicing veterinarian who deals with new puppy owners' questions and concerns on a daily basis. I've tried to cover as many topics as possible; ideas for what to include in the book have come from the numerous questions, comments, and suggestions often posed by new puppy owners. An important part of this book is the discussion concerning what it costs to raise a puppy and how to afford the care a new puppy requires. While this information might discourage some of you from owning a puppy, my intention is to better prepare you for those unexpected expenses that invariably arise after purchasing that new puppy.

Puppies are fun and playful and bring a smile to our faces. Enjoy your new puppy, and do a good job raising him. When you need advice, don't hesitate to turn to *Your Puppy's First Year* for answers.

Chapter 1
Choosing a Puppy

Choosing a puppy seems easy enough. You just decide if you want a male or female, go to the local pet shop, spend several hundred dollars, and pick the cutest puppy in the window. You take it home, provide it nutrition, love, and regular veterinary care. It never gets sick and lives to a ripe old age. Ah, if only life were so easy.

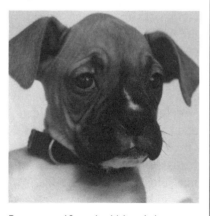

Bronwyn, a 10-week-old female boxer

Choosing a puppy is a difficult job. Unfortunately, so many people make an impulse buy based on emotion, only to find out the puppy is sick, has behavioral problems, or costs a lot in upkeep. These poor puppies, chosen on the spur of the moment, often end up euthanized before their third birthday. It is estimated that 12 to 20 million dogs and cats are euthanized in animal shelters each year. Careful planning for a new puppy can prevent many of these needless deaths.

Pets are not disposable items. It takes time to evaluate your reasons for wanting a dog and then decide on the right one.

Ideally, you should choose and then visit with a veterinarian *before* purchasing a puppy. Veterinarians are trained to help you

1

decide if a puppy is for you and can help you decide which breed may best suit you. Finally, the veterinarian can give you a realistic idea of the care and the expense involved in caring for this pet over the next 10-20 years.

Choosing a veterinarian is discussed in detail in Chapter 2.

Why Do You Want a Puppy?

This is an extremely important question all potential puppy owners should ponder before buying their puppy. What are your reasons for wanting a puppy? Companionship? Status? A playmate for the kids? Do you want a "pet quality" puppy or a "breeding" or "show" quality puppy?

What Breed to Choose?

What breed you pick is dependent upon several factors.

• •➡ If you live in a small space such as an apartment, obviously a large breed such as a Doberman pinscher or Labrador retriever is not for you.

• •➡ If you like a lot of physical activity, such as jogging, a lap breed like a Maltese would not fit your lifestyle.

• •➡ If you want a breed that doesn't shed, a poodle or Bichon frise is better for you than a retriever or cocker spaniel.

• •➡ If grooming is something you don't want to deal with, a Bichon frise or poodle is not for you.

Purebred dogs are prone to breed-specific problems. That's not to say that every member of that breed will develop a problem, only that dogs of a particular breed have a higher chance of contracting a specific problem than the general dog population. As a rule, mixed breeds (muts) are usually sturdier and less likely to develop problems than purebred dogs.

It is beyond the scope of this book to mention every breed and its problems; your veterinarian can assist you with that, as can the American Kennel Club (AKC) dog book found in most libraries. Some generalizations can be made:

• •➡ Large dogs, such as golden and Labrador retrievers, collies, Great Danes, and German shepherds, have a higher incidence of musculoskeletal diseases than smaller breeds.

• •➡ Poodles and cocker spaniels have a higher incidence of ear and eye diseases.

••➡ Retrievers and terriers have a higher incidence of allergic skin diseases and eye diseases than other breeds.

••➡ Small breeds of dogs are commonly afflicted with valvular heart disease as they age; large breeds are more prone to cardiomyopathy, a serious illness, leading to failure of the heart.

Puppy or Adult?

Okay, so you've decided a dog is definitely for you. After careful study and discussion with your veterinarian, you've even made a decision about which breed may best suit you. Now you have to decide if a young puppy or older dog is what you want.

While puppies can be fine pets, so too can the older ones. Remember that puppies require a

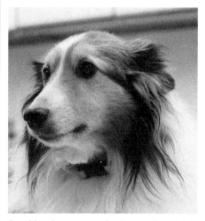

An older dog may easier to care for and may already be housebroken.

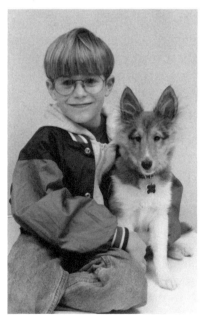

A puppy can be a great companion for children.

lot of work and expense their first year. If you don't have the time or don't want to go to the trouble and expense of puppy care, you should seriously consider adopting an older pet, especially one that may be at the local pound. Many of these dogs are purebred pets (although without papers), and most if not all of them will make excellent pets.

Breed rescue clubs (ask your veterinarian for names and

telephone numbers) also have purebred dogs available, usually for a very low cost. These dogs are placed in foster homes prior to adoption and usually make excellent pets, as dogs with diseases are not offered for sale or for adoption.

Here are some points to ponder when deciding between a young puppy or older dog.

●●➡ Puppies must be housetrained; older dogs usually are already housetrained.

●●➡ Puppies must be vaccinated, dewormed, and spayed or neutered; many older pets have already had these procedures performed (although all dogs need physical exams, vaccinations, and other veterinary care annually).

●●➡ Puppies bite and chew everything in sight; most older dogs do not have destructive chewing problems.

●●➡ Most puppies have not developed behavioral problems (other than biting and chewing); some older dogs may have behavioral problems.

●●➡ You can train your puppy the way you want; you and you alone will determine what kind of pet it will become. An older dog has already been trained by another owner. It may have been left at the pound because the owner mistrained it as a puppy and now it is an older dog with behavioral problems that its former owner could not handle.

●●➡ Many puppies have medical problems including worms (parasites), fleas, ear mites, or kennel cough; most older dogs are healthy (although they may harbor intestinal parasites or

---

TEETHING. . . . .

Puppies go through a "teething" phase, just like children. Until 6 months of age, when most or all of the adult teeth have erupted, your puppy will gradually lose his baby teeth. Unlike in children, the procedure is usually not painful and often goes unnoticed. Puppies usually do not act irritable, get diarrhea, or develop a fever as new teeth erupt. However, teething puppies usually need to chew on something. You can help them out by offering a variety of chew toys as suggested by your veterinarian.

MONTHLY PET HEALTH
CHECKLIST

New puppies owners are often overly concerned about their puppy's health. An occasional cough or sneeze, one mild bout of vomiting or diarrhea, and an occasional scratch are not usually cause for concern. Your puppy is not that different from you. Since you wouldn't call the doctor if you coughed a few times, there is no reason to panic if your puppy also exhibits an occasional mild symptom.

There are times when you should be concerned. Persistent vomiting, diarrhea, coughing, sneezing, itching, or lack of appetite or energy are reasons to call the doctor. The following home health checklist, which should be used monthly, can help you decide if your puppy requires veterinary attention.

Answer "yes" or "no" to the following questions. Call your doctor if you answer "yes" to any of the questions.

My puppy....
walks with pain or difficulty.
has abnormal feces.
urinates abnormally.
has an abnormal appetite; eats or drinks too much or too little.
vomits.
has difficulty breathing.
has offensive breath odor.
does not have clean white teeth and pink healthy gums.
has lumps or bumps on its body.
has ticks or fleas or ear mites.
shakes his head.
licks, chews, bites at, or scratches himself constantly.
has hair loss or abnormal-looking skin.
passes out or tires easily.
has discharge from the eyes, nose, mouth, anus, or genitals.

heartworms and should be checked for these conditions).

•••➡ Some puppies may have congenital conditions, such as hip or elbow dysplasia, that may not be apparent until they get a little older; older dogs have usually had time to show any signs of congenital diseases.

•••➡ Puppies are fun and playful; it is a joy to watch them explore and learn about their environment; older dogs have already experienced this energetic time of "puppyhood."

While it may appear that the odds are stacked in favor of purchasing an older dog, that's not really true. There are positive and negative benefits about owning either a puppy or older dog. As a prospective owner, you need to make an informed decision. If you can handle all the challenges of puppyhood, you will be rewarded with much happiness watching that puppy grow and mature and live a long, healthy life.

Common Owner Concerns

Q: I have several small children and we are considering purchasing a puppy for them. Are there any breeds I should avoid? We certainly don't want to pick a puppy that will be aggressive and bite the children as it gets older.

A: I would warn you never to buy a puppy for the sole reason of buying it for "the kids." Most children cannot handle the total responsibility of caring for a puppy. Also, keep in mind that there is no one breed that is best for every situation. However, there are some general points

to consider in choosing a breed:

If you can see both the mother and father of the puppies, and they are friendly and outgoing, especially around children, your puppy will most likely inherit these desirable behaviors as well.

Regarding dog bites, the following breeds were the most common to be reported to state agencies, hospitals, and veterinary behaviorists: chow chow, pit bull, German shepherd, Rottweiler, Labrador and golden retriever, Doberman pinscher, cocker spaniel, and springer spaniel. Many veterinarians have experiences which differ slightly from these reports: As a rule, the smaller breeds (Chihuahua, Lhasa apso, Shih Tzu), seem to be more likely to bite children (and also the veterinary staff!) than most of the larger breeds. While retrievers are often mentioned in bite risk studies, most of the larger dogs (including retrievers) are excellent family dogs.

Once again, if both parent dogs are friendly around children, chances are the puppy you select will be as well. How a puppy turns out depends quite a bit on genetics, but it also depends on the way you raise it. For this reason, it's critical that owners get the proper instructions on behavior management from their doctors. The breeder who sells you your new puppy should also discuss any potential behavioral (and medical) problems with your puppy's breed. All puppies should be enrolled with their owners in puppy training classes that are reinforced with additional classes as the puppy reaches 6-12 months of age. Families with children may

VACATION FOR YOUR PUPPY . . . .

While you're away on vacation, your puppy can "vacation" at your veterinarian's hospital in the boarding area (kennel). Some owners are concerned about how their pet will fare while they are away. Most pets do well during their boarding visit. Prior to boarding your pet, make sure it's current on all its vaccinations. It's also a good idea for you to see the kennel and make sure you are comfortable with it. Ask about ventilation and heating and air-conditioning. Find out how often pets are walked, what brand of food is fed and how often, and what happens in case of an emergency.

While many owners like to leave a favorite toy or bedding with the puppy, many facilities discourage this practice. While it doesn't happen often, a boarding pet could destroy a toy and swallow a piece which might cause an injury. For this reason, it's safer not to leave anything for the puppy. Most boarding puppies don't even play with any of the toys that owners leave for them. While it may make you feel better, the puppy does fine without the toys.

want to avoid purchasing an older dog (unless the dog is familiar and known to enjoy children) since there is no way to tell if it was socialized with children or how the previous owners raised it. Larger breeds tend to be more tolerant of children pulling tails and ears and roughhousing with the dogs, whereas smaller breeds seem to be more aggressive in these situations. Bites from larger breeds, especially pit bulls (which are usually nice dogs to people but not so nice to other dogs), are usually more serious due to the size difference between the dog and the child and the jaw strength of the dog.

To prevent dog bites, puppies should be disciplined for biting, biting games and tug-of-war games should be discouraged, and all people in the house should be taught the proper methods of reward and punishment. All house members should discipline the puppy for unacceptable behaviors. Dogs should be neutered or spayed to prevent hormone-induced aggression. Puppies should be conditioned to allow or to permit all family members to remove food or toys without showing signs of aggression. Small children should be trained not to approach dogs

without parental assistance (many bites are precipitated when the child approaches a dog, even a friend's dog, and displays what the dog considers a threatening gesture, as when the child may grab for the dog, its food, or toys). Finally, small children should never be left alone with a dog, especially the larger breeds which are strong and can play pretty hard.

Aggression in dogs can usually be successfully treated when working with a veterinarian knowledgeable in animal behavior. Your veterinarian may use a combination of drug therapy and a behavior modifying training program (often working with a responsible trainer) to treat aggression. Behavior modification takes time and can be expensive. Behavior problems, especially those involving aggression, are best prevented.

Q: Where should I acquire a puppy? Is one source better than another?

A: Ideally, if you can see the mother and father of the puppies in person, this is a great situation. If the parent dogs exhibit any undesirable behaviors, such as aggression or excessive timidity, this can be observed. If the parents have any medical or physical characteristics which might be passed to the puppies, this may also be determined. If both parents seem in excellent health and physical shape and do not exhibit any undesirable behaviors, you can be reasonably certain the puppies will also be of the same high quality.

While many people feel that pet stores are the worst places to buy puppies, a recent study failed to reveal a significant increase of illness in puppies from pet stores. Here's some of what the study, as reported in the June 15, 1994 issue of the *Journal of the American Veterinary Medical Association*, had to say:

1. The risk of acquiring a fatally ill pup is low regardless of where it is acquired (breeder, pet store, humane society).

CLEAN TEETH MEAN A HEALTHY BODY ....

Dental disease is the #1 disease of dogs 3 years of age and older. Brushing your pet's teeth at home will decrease the number of visits (and the cost!) for professional cleaning (which is usually needed on average once a year). The most important thing you can do for your puppy is *daily* brushing of his teeth. All you need is a soft-bristled child's toothbrush and some water. Spend only about 5-10 seconds several times each day and gently brush the outside surfaces of the teeth (it's almost impossible to get any pet to let you brush the inner surfaces). Brush as you would your own teeth. Avoid human toothpaste or baking soda and hydrogen peroxide as they can foam up in the pet's mouth and make the experience unpleasant. Most puppies think of the brushing as a game and easily accept it. Training your puppy to accept tooth brushing not only controls dental disease but trains him to allow you to do an important procedure without a struggle.

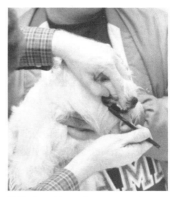

Daily brushing of your puppy's teeth controls periodontal disease and only takes a few seconds of your time.

2. The risk of respiratory disease is higher for pups obtained from pet stores, but serious disease is rare and doesn't differ significantly between sources. The stress of weaning, shipping, handling, and exposure to other puppies increases their risk.

3. Puppies from humane societies had the second highest incidence of respiratory disease, followed by those acquired from breeders and finally private owners.

4. Regardless of source, pups 10-12 weeks old had the highest risk of respiratory disease.

5. Puppies from humane societies and pet stores had the highest incidence of intestinal disease; severe disease was rare regardless of source of acquisition. As with respiratory disease, stresses associated with weaning, shipping, handling, and mixing puppies contributed to intestinal disease.

6. Puppies purchased from private owners had the highest incidence of roundworms, a disease that can be fatal in puppies if not detected and treated early. This disease can also be contracted from puppies by owners.

7. Puppies acquired from pet stores had a low prevalence of intestinal parasites due to routine deworming programs.

8. Flea control was better in pet stores pups than those bought from private owners or the humane societies.

9. Puppies from breeders and pet stores had a higher incidence of ear mites.

10. Seven to 15 percent of puppies have some type of congenital defects.

These findings indicate that regardless of source, the risk of death and serious illness was low. However, some pet stores and breeders do not properly socialize their puppies and may sell puppies with behavioral problems. Be sure to ask the seller what type of socializing has been done to the puppy.

There is no ideal source from which to acquire a puppy. The decision is up to the individual owner after considering all factors. Obviously, if you are not impressed with the seller or the facilities or quality of puppies, you should not try to be a "Good Samaritan" and purchase a puppy from that source. Puppies that are ill and which require veterinary care can be expensive to treat and may die depending upon the type of disease present.

While it is ideal to be able to see the parents of the puppy, it is not essential for picking a happy, healthy puppy. Make sure the puppy is friendly, outgoing, and seems physically fit. Regardless of where you purchase the puppy, insist on a guarantee in your written contract that allows you to return the puppy if a veterinarian finds any major health problems; have the puppy examined as soon after purchase as possible, ideally within 24 to 48 hours.

Q: Is it true that small dogs live longer than large dogs?

A: A recent study reported in *Veterinary Medicine* magazine did confirm this long-held belief. Giant breeds (Saint Bernard, Great Dane, Irish wolfhound) had a significantly greater risk of developing heart, musculoskeletal, skin, and cancerous diseases. Small breeds (under 20 pounds) had a higher chance of developing disease of the nervous, endocrine, and urogenital systems. The risk of musculoskeletal diseases in giant breeds increased with age. Heart disease was higher in giant breeds 4-7 years of age whereas it was greater in small dogs over 10 years of age. Giant breeds

were more likely affected with cancer before 10 years of age. The highest rate of death in giant breeds occurred in the 4-7-year-old age group; few of these dogs live to 10 years of age. A significant number of small breed dogs lived more than 10 years. As a generalization, giant breeds live about 8 years, large breeds live about 10-12 years, and small breeds live 12-15 years. Increased longevity is definitely linked to proper veterinary care, early disease diagnosis, and prompt treatment.

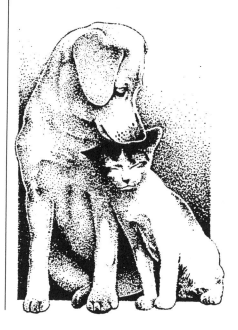

Are We Soul Mates?
· ·

A Guide for Selecting the Correct Dog for Your Needs

Not all dogs are suited for all people (and vice versa). Some people should never own a dog of any kind, any time!

From Your Childhood:

Did you, your family, or close friend own a dog?

What are your memories of this dog?

What was its size, type, length of hair?

Who fed, exercised, and cared for this dog?

Was this dog trained? By whom?

What is your last memory of this dog?

How old was the dog when you last remember it? How old were you?

Do you have good memories or bad memories of this dog?

Had this dog's physical activity lessened as it matured?

Was it more or less troublesome in its old age?

Do you remember this dog as a young, wild, active, undiciplined puppy?

Are You Prepared for a New Dog?

Where will the dog sleep and eat?

How many hours per day will it be alone?

Where will the puppy be kept in the house?

Who will be responsible for feeding, exercise, cleaning up after it, and taking it to the doctor?

Who will pay for its upkeep (food, toys, grooming, behavior classes, veterinary bills)?

Do you have a fenced yard, pen, or dog run?

Will you spend the money to build one?

Will a new dog get along with present pets?

Have you selected a reputable veterinarian, groomer, and trainer?

Have you asked the veterinarian about fees for: office visits, medications, immunizations, spaying/neutering, long term medications for older pets with diabetes, epilepsy, or cancer?

Who will housetrain the new puppy?

Are you familiar with dog crates?

Do you think it is cruel to place a puppy or dog "in a box"?

Have you recently installed new carpeting or acquired expensive furniture?

Have you considered a dog that is already housetrained?

If you travel, who will take care of the pet in your absence?

Have you read any books or consulted with your veterinarian about dogs in general or specific breeds?

Have you discussed the pros and cons of various breeds with a knowledgeable, objective person who is not in the business of selling dogs?

Have you read books about dog behavior and early puppy development?

Are you familiar with the Promise management system dog collar (at $40-$50)?

Puppy Assessment

A dog's personality needs to match your own personality and lifestyle. What do you feel is the most important characteristic for your dog?

Who will spend the most time with your dog?

Do you want a puppy that is robust, playful, and full of energy?

Do you want a puppy that craves attention, wanting and needing to be physically close to you constantly?

Do you want a puppy that wants to cuddle and be held in your lap?

Do you prefer a dog who is independent and leaves you alone?

Will your dog live indoors, outdoors, or both?

What will you do with your dog during the day?

Do you live close to neighbors who might object to a barking dog?

Do you have a securely fenced backyard?

Do you care if your dog digs in the yard?

Do you have an expensive garden that your pet might destroy?

Do you want a dog to be friendly to neighbors, your children, their children, and your children's playmates?

Do you engage in outdoor recreational activities such as camping, hunting, or fishing? Do you want your dog to accompany you on these trips?

Physical Appearance

Do you prefer small dogs, medium dogs, or giant dogs?

Do you want a dog with a lot of hair? Some breeds require regular grooming, most require daily brushing and at least occasional bathing, and many shed excessively all year (although this can often be controlled, see Chapter 7).

Does a breed that requires less upkeep sound more appealing?

Are you aware that larger breeds generally have a shorter lifespan than small breeds?

Training

Who will be responsible for the dog's manners?

Do you have the patience to train your dog?

Do you agree on the importance of training your dog?

How much time and money will you devote to proper training?

Is it important that you have a breed that is relatively easy to train?

Are you prepared to be the "alpha"dog in the household?

Do you have the confidence to live with a strong-willed breed?

Will other family members (children) be dominant to the pet?

Children

Do you have children?

Do the children know the difference between a dog, as a living creature, and a furry "toy"?

Will your dog be around children a lot?

Would a mature, already housetrained dog be easier for you to manage at this time?

Do you believe that children can be intentionally cruel to a puppy and cause it harm?

Is acquiring this puppy something you are doing "for the children"?

Protection

Are you getting the dog for protection? Why?

Do you want the dog to bark and alert you? Will the neighbors object?

Do you plan to invest the necessary time and money in training your dog to be a guard dog?

Have you checked local zoning codes regarding guard dogs?

Are you prepared to face the legal/financial complications and responsibilities of owning a guard dog?

Have you discussed this with your attorney and insurance company?

Male or Female

Do you have a prefenence for male or female? Why?

Are you planning to show your dog? Can you afford the expense of traveling the country for entering the pet in shows?

Are you considering a male dog to avoid heat cycles and pregnancies?

Are you familiar with the behavioral and medical differences of male and female dogs?

Are you planning to breed your dog? Can you afford to breed your dog? Do you know what is involved in being an ethical breeder?

Are you planning to spay or neuter your pet? Do you know the benefits of spaying and neutering?

Do you know the behavioral and medical problems (such as cancer) that can occur in dogs that are not spayed or neutered?

Dealing with a Breeder

Definitions:

Breeder: An individual who owns a female dog and allows it to have a litter of puppies.

Backyard Breeder: An inexperienced individual who happens to own a purebred dog and breeds it to another purebred dog without any knowledge of genetics and without any interest in bettering the breed.

Hobby Breeder: An individual having a registered litter to better the breed. Usually part of the hobby of training/showing dogs.

Commercial Breeder: Individual owning many registered females, producing many litters and puppies for financial gain, often called "puppy mills."

What is the breeder's reason for having this litter of puppies?

Do the puppies live in a clean area? Are the mother and father of the puppies friendly, clean, and healthy?

Are the mother and father dog bred to each other often?

Is this a planned litter?

How many litters does the mother have each year? How old is she, and how many litters has she had in her life?

Can you visit the puppies from previous litters?

Can you contact other owners for their recommendations?

Is the breeder willing to stand behind the puppy and give a written guarantee for health and inherited or congenital problems?

Will the breeder replace the puppy if you are not happy with it or if it gets sick? Will the breeder give a refund?

What about inherited orthopedic or eye problems that may not show up for several years?

Do the mother and father dog have allergies or health problems? Can you contact their veterinarian to be sure?

Does the breeder do her own vaccinations and dewormings?

Have the puppies been checked by a veterinarian? Why not?

Do relatives of the puppy have any health problems (cancer, allergies, orthopedic or eye disorders, heart or other organ disorders)?

Did the breeder have a veterinarian take radiographs (X-rays) or do an opthalmic (eye) exam on the parents prior to breeding? If so, can she prove it? If not, why not?

Was any pre-breeding genetic testing performed? Why not?

Has the breeder done any puppy personality testing? Why not?

If you are looking at the last remaining puppy in the litter, why wasn't this one selected earlier? Was he sick? Is she shy or aggressive (a fear biter)?

Did the breeder volunteer references? If not, what was his reaction when you asked?
Have you checked out the references?

Registration with any kennel club, such as the AKC (American Kennel Club), is not a sign of a quality animal. Registration is simply that; the dogs are on file with the club after the breeder pays a registration fee. "Papers" are meaningless and are not a sign of a quality animal.

The preceding information was reprinted from a handout used by Margaret Fitch, a dog trainer we recommend to all of our new puppy owners. The questions posed give you more food for thought when deciding if you should own a pet. We appreciate Mrs. Fitch letting us reprint this information for your use and for her help in the preparation of this book.

Chapter 2

Choosing
Your Puppy's Doctor

· ·

Choosing a veterinarian is an extremely important job for pet owners. As with choosing the family doctor or dentist, choosing a veterinarian for the new puppy shouldn't be left to chance or done on a whim. Remember, this person will most likely be providing health care for your four-legged family member for many years. You need to choose someone you trust, someone you can develop a rapport with, someone who shares the same health care philosophy with you, and someone who is convenient and offers high-quality, affordable care.

The best time to choose a veterinarian is *before* you ever purchase your puppy. Your veterinarian can help you make the right choice in a pet. Maybe a puppy isn't for you; possibly a kitten would be a better match for your situation. If a puppy is the way to go, which breed should you choose? Your veterinarian can give you advice on proper selection after meeting with you and your family and finding out your interests.

You should plan on taking your new puppy to the doctor very soon after purchasing it, ideally the same day. Most sellers, including pet stores and breeders, give owners five to seven days to have their puppy examined. Some sellers stipulate that the puppy must be examined within 48 hours of purchase. If the puppy isn't examined within the stipulated time frame, the

buyer's contract and health guarantee is voided. This means that
if the puppy isn't examined
within the stated time after purchase, the treatment of any
problems or diseases detected by
the doctor are the owner's
responsibility. Within the terms
of the contract, an owner whose
puppy is found to have a problem within the stated time frame
will be compensated by the
seller. Let's say for example that
you take your puppy to the veterinarian the day it is purchased.
During the initial exam, the
doctor discovers ear mites, a relatively common problem in new
puppies. Diagnosis and treatment for ear mites might be
$50-$60. Because the puppy was
examined while it was still
"under warranty," you are reimbursed in full by the seller. Had
you waited a week or more, you
would not be reimbursed for the
cost of the ear mite treatment.

Of course this is just an
example, and every seller will
have different conditions in the
warranty (make sure you ask for
and receive a warranty or written
contract with your new puppy!).
The point is that once the puppy
is purchased, you don't have
time to visit several veterinarians
and try to choose the right one
for you. You must be comfortable with your decision; spend
the time looking around *before*
you buy the puppy.

Choosing a doctor for your
pet is serious business, and it's a
task that should not be taken
lightly. Ask friends or family
members to recommend a
veterinarian, or call the local
veterinary association (the phone
number is usually available in
the yellow pages under the
"veterinary" listing). After
compiling a list of prospective or
possible veterinarians, it's time
to do some investigating. If you
follow the procedures listed
below, you should have no problem narrowing your selection to
that one "perfect" veterinarian.

••➡ **Call the office and ask
questions.** You want to find out
how the staff treats you on the
phone. A rude or uncaring atti-
tude is an indication of how
you'll be treated in the office.
Since you'll be doing most of
your business with the staff and
not the doctor, it's imperative
that you are satisfied with them.
Of course, everyone has a bad
day at one time or another. So if
you are treated rudely on the
phone, you may want to try a
second call or choose another
veterinarian from your
remaining list of names.

Some questions to ask during your telephone inquiry:

1. What vaccinations and other services does my puppy need?
2. What is the cost for those services?
3. What are the office hours?
4. What forms of payment are accepted?
5. Are clients billed? (To keep costs down, most veterinarians don't bill.)
6. Does the veterinarian take emergency calls? (Most don't.)

The answers to these questions, are not as important as *how* they are answered. A staff member who can't comfortably answer these questions might be indicative of an overall problem (poorly trained staff) at the office. Make sure you're comfortable with how you are treated on the phone.

••➡ **Visit the office.** If you're happy with the way you have been treated on the phone, ask to visit the office. Any office should allow you to stop by for a

---

AFTER HOURS VETERINARY CARE . . . .

Most veterinarians do not take emergency calls. However, pets often get sick after hours and require immediate care. Many cities have animal emergency clinics for after-hours treatment.

While emergency clinics can literally be life-savers, you need to be aware of several things. First, because they are emergency clinics, you should avoid using them for routine problems; go instead to your regular veterinarian. Second, because of the overhead cost, expect to pay more for this specialized care. Third, because they offer strictly temporary care, you will probably still need to go to your regular veterinarian the next day.

If you're not sure if you have a true emergency, call the clinic and ask their advice. If you need to go, call ahead so the staff can give you instructions and prepare for your arrival. Ask your own doctor the name, address, and phone number of the emergency clinic he uses and keep the number handy. Finally, don't put off minor problems until they become big problems (usually on the weekends or holidays) that require emergency care.

quick tour and possible introduction to the doctor. An office that refuses a tour may have something to hide: *beware*! Realize that certain times may be busy or inconvenient for the staff, however, and work with them to arrange a mutually satisfactory time.

••➡ **Look, listen, and, most importantly, smell.** Is the parking area clean, safe, and close to the office? You don't want to have to walk far with a pet that might get loose or expose your pet to unsafe conditions. Does the office appear and smell clean? While occasional "accidents" on the floor do occur, a dirty or smelly office might indicate that the place is not kept clean and sanitary, certainly not a place you want your pet to visit. Is the staff warm and courteous in person as well as on the phone? Do you get to see everything, including the boarding area, surgical facilities, and treatment rooms? If you don't feel comfortable in the office, neither will your pet; look elsewhere.

••➡ **Meet the doctor.** Most doctors will be glad to meet a prospective client for a few minutes at no charge. Don't be afraid to ask the doctor any questions you have, such as:

1. Where and when did you receive your degree?
2. How long have you been in practice?
3. Do you have any specialized interests (birds, dermatology, surgery, etc.)?
4. Do you treat clients with after-hours emergencies or refer them to a reputable facility?
5. Do you have any pets of your own?
6. When is your day off, and who fills in when you are gone?
7. Do you feel pets should be spayed or neutered, and at what age?

As you question the doctor, notice *how* the questions are answered. You should feel comfortable with the doctor and the staff. Remember, you will be entrusting your pet's care to this person for possibly 15-20 years.

••➡ **Price … Quality … Service. Pick any two.** I've heard this saying many times, and it's so true. If you want a low price, you usually have to give up high quality or superior service. As you make calls to schedule visits with the various offices, you'll probably find a wide range of answers to questions about the price of services. For example, some veterinarians may charge $50 for the first puppy visit, whereas others charge $20. Some doctors may charge $120 to spay a pet; another doctor might quote you $30! What's going on here? Are you being ripped off?

Probably not; the difference in price is related to the difference in the quality of care and the level of customer service you receive.

For example, the average new puppy visit at my office takes 30-60 minutes. We feel justified in charging a higher

MALPRACTICE ....

Most veterinarians don't have the malpractice worries that "people doctors" face on a daily basis. However, since anyone can file a lawsuit, no matter how frivolous, at any time, veterinarians must always strive to prevent problems from occurring.

By definition, malpractice must involve an action that a veterinarian takes (or fails to take) that another veterinarian of reasonable judgement would not have taken (or would have taken if needed) that results in measurable harm or death to the patient.

As an example, if your healthy puppy dies after a spaying procedure, is that malpractice? It all depends. Assuming the doctor performed the surgery as another doctor of similar skill would have, even though the puppy died there was no malpractice. However, if that doctor administered the incorrect dose of anesthetic, this would possibly be malpractice.

Let's suppose that a doctor accidentally left a surgical sponge in your puppy's abdomen after a spay. Even though that is negligent and not normal procedure, unless your puppy suffered from it (developed an infection or died as a direct result of the sponge), no malpractice was committed since no harm was done.

Remember, for malpractice to occur there must be a negligent action or inaction *and* measurable harm must occur as a direct result of the negligent act.

price for the time we will take, thoroughly examining the pet, teaching the owner how to be a responsible puppy owner, explaining diet and training, laying the foundation for a life of proper health care, and answering questions. Lower-cost facilities may rush clients in and out in an effort to see as many as possible. Make sure your veterinarian administers only the best vaccinations, always using a new needle and syringe (some places actually give vaccinations with used, but supposedly "resterilized," needles and syringes).

Common Owner Concerns...

Word-of-Mouth Referrals

Q: My next door neighbor raved about her veterinarian. Is he the one I should choose for my new puppy?

A: From the doctor's viewpoint, clients who choose them because of word-of-mouth referrals are often their best clients. If one client is satisfied, he or she will likely refer friends. These new clients are usually also outstanding clients.

While getting suggestions from friends is a great way to gather a few names for your list, it is still necessary to actually do some investigative work on your own. Just because your friend likes a certain doctor and his policies doesn't mean that you will. Think of friends as a great starting place for names to add to your list of prospective doctors.

Choosing a Doctor from the Phone Book

Q: The yellow pages seem like a convenient way to find a doctor. Is there anything I should worry about when choosing a doctor from the phone book?

A: While the yellow pages are used by people for many things, most people don't choose a doctor from this source. The research I did for a marketing book for veterinarians showed that, on average, only about 7 percent of new clients came from the yellow pages. The yellow pages can be helpful to select a few doctors in a certain location, however. Let's say that you don't want to go more than five miles from your home for a veterinarian. Using the phone book, you can pick out veterinary offices near you to add to your list of prospective veterinarians.

One note of caution: Don't believe everything you read! Realize that as with any source of advertising, ads in the phone book are meant to attract your attention and get you to respond. Not everything in an ad is necessarily true and accurate. For example, some doctors advertise that they treat birds. While they may offer treatment for birds, it doesn't necessarily mean they know what they are doing! Use the ads as a source, but don't be over-impressed with what you read. If something sounds too good to be true, it usually is!

Driving in the Neighborhood

Q: I pass several clinics driving to work each day. They all are convenient for me. How do I decide which one is best?

A: Many people choose a veterinarian because they have seen the office and its location is convenient. That's not the best way to choose a veterinarian, but it is helpful in compiling your list of possible choices. The only way you can ultimately decide which

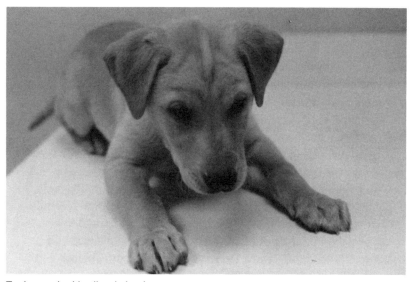

Twelve-week-old yellow Labrador puppy

doctor is best for your pet is by calling and then visiting the office. After some investigative work, you will be able to decide which doctor best suits your needs.

Differences in Costs

Q: I've called several offices and it seems like there is quite a range in the costs for vaccinations. Why do some doctors charge more than others for the same shots?

A: In the competitive environment in which we live, it's no surprise that discount pet clinics have appeared on the scene. In order to hook you as a client, a clinic may offer cut-rate prices (and corresponding cut-rate care) to lure you in. As a client, you and you alone have to make a choice regarding the care for

---

AN OWNER'S RESPONSIBILITY . . . .

Neither in human nor veterinary medicine can a guaranteed cure ever be offered. While we can always do our best to cure a problem, there are too many factors involved that doctors can't control to ever promise a certain outcome. What if the outcome is not as expected? What if your pet dies during what should be a "routine" procedure? What is your responsibility?

You may be surprised to discover that legally you are required to pay for all requested services regardless of the outcome. Let's suppose that your "normal" puppy dies after what seemed to be a routine spay surgery. Are you still responsible for payment? Yes. The reason is because no guarantee as to the outcome of the procedure was given. You requested a spay, and even though the surgery resulted in the unfortunate death of your puppy, you are still responsible for payment for the services you requested.

No doctor can ever guarantee any treatment or surgery, and no procedure or surgery should ever be considered "routine." While extremely uncommon, there are rare instances of normal-appearing pets dying during or after properly performed medical and surgical procedures. Know the risks of the procedure before making the decision to schedule the surgery.

your new puppy. Do you want high-quality care or low-cost care? There is no right or wrong, only choices—choices you make and you will have to live with once you make your decision.

Hospital or Clinic

Q. Some veterinary offices are called "hospitals" whereas others are called "clinics." What's the difference?

A. Often, very little. As of this writing, veterinarians can choose whatever names they want for their offices. The terms "hospital" and "clinic" are interchangeable. Many doctors feel that the term "hospital" sounds more professional than "clinic," and some hospitals do offer more services than clinics offer.

Is Low Cost Really Worth It?

Q: Why do some doctors offer low-cost neutering and spaying, whereas others charge two to three times as much?

A: Regarding spays and neuters, the higher price usually includes additional services, such as a pre-surgical examination and blood tests to make sure it's safe to anesthetize your pet. For example, after the exam and blood tests the veterinarian may then sedate the animal, which reduces the amount of anesthetic needed, making the procedure safer. The veterinarian may use isoflurane, a very expensive anesthetic gas, but also the safest. A more expensive suture material may be used for the stitches which helps reduce infection and swelling after the surgery, and your pet may be monitored during the surgery by an assistant as well as various machines. Post-operative care is also a factor.

Consequently you may be cutting the quality of your pet's care by cutting costs. You as the owner must decide if cost or quality will be the driving factor in choosing a veterinarian for your pet. For tips on cutting costs without sacrificing care, see Chapter 13, "Lowering the Cost of Pet Care."

GETTING A SECOND OPINION . . . .

Most pet owners are happy with their doctors. Unless a problem arises, a pet owner has little reason to seek the opinion of another veterinarian. But what if you're not happy with your doctor? What if, despite his best recommendations, your puppy continues to be sick and not improve? What can you do?

Before you jump ship, consider asking your veterinarian *why* he thinks the problem isn't getting better. Could the diagnosis or treatment be incorrect? Could your pet be one of those rare ones that doesn't respond to the "usual" treatment for the disease?

Be honest with yourself as well. Do you have anything to do with your pet not improving? For example, are you giving your pet the medicine exactly as prescribed by the doctor? So often the reason for a pet not getting better or getting better and then relapsing is that the owner is not giving all of the medication as prescribed. Have you placed any financial constraints on the doctor? If you declined any tests that may be necessary to accurately diagnose and treat your pet, chances are your pet may never get better! The more information you give your doctor (by agreeing to his recommendations for diagnostic testing and treatment), the greater the chance for a correct diagnosis and treatment.

If you still feel a second opinion is needed, there's nothing wrong with that. You can assist the new doctor if you bring copies of your previous medical records. I suggest a second opinion if your pet has had a chronic problem for several months and is not improving despite the fact that your regular doctor has tried several different treatments and you have not placed financial constraints on him. Getting a second opinion will, as a rule, cost more than a first opinion. Be prepared to agree to extensive diagnostic testing in order for the new doctor to give you an honest and valuable second opinion.

Chapter 3
Vaccinations

● ●

A̲n important part of health care for your puppy is a series of shots, or vaccinations. These vaccinations occur in a series that will be repeated throughout the life of the pet.

Vaccinations are an inexpensive way to protect your pet from the common diseases that are easily transmitted between other dogs and your pet.

There are several reasons to have your pet properly immunized:

●●➡ Regular vaccinations are the least expensive way to prevent common diseases.

●●➡ Vaccinations are the only way to prevent certain fatal diseases.

●●➡ Vaccinations are required before your puppy can be boarded, groomed, or hospitalized.

●●➡ Having your pet vaccinated demonstrates your responsibility as a loving, caring pet owner.

Most of the time, you will choose to have your puppy vaccinated at your regular veterinarian's office. There are two other options that you may hear about, however. Both of these options are inferior to visiting your regular doctor and can jeopardize not only your pet's health but its life and your health as well.

Vaccination Clinics. Mobile, parking-lot shot clinics are a common sight in many communities. At these clinics, low-cost vaccinations are given in a conveyor-belt fashion. While these shots do usually cost less than those at your regular doctor's, *buyer beware*! There are many negative aspects about these clinics:

1. While they charge less than a full-service hospital, they don't charge that much less (usually $5-$10 less at most).

2. You may pay less, but you also get less. The cost of the vaccination probably does not include a fecal exam for parasites or a thorough physical exam. While vaccinations are extremely important, the exam is even more important. Why? Think about it: how many pets do you personally know that have died from rabies or distemper? Very few if any. Yet, how many pets die each year of kidney, liver, or heart failure, or cancer? Many. The only way to accurately diagnose these common conditions is with a yearly examination and appropriate laboratory tests. While vaccinations are important, so is the physical examination; don't put your pet's health at risk just to save a few dollars.

3. At low-cost shot clinics, your puppy is not an individual but rather a number. Maintaining a regular relationship with one doctor is important in establishing continuity of care.

4. At the low-cost clinics, your puppy will be exposed to all the other pets standing in line, waiting for the shots. You have no way of knowing if any of these other pets are current on their vaccinations. More than likely they are not; many have never had any vaccinations (some studies have found that up to half of the pets at the "shot clinics" do not receive regular veterinary care!). By taking your puppy to its regular doctor, you will limit its exposure to unvaccinated animals.

5. Vaccinations are required for boarding, grooming, and

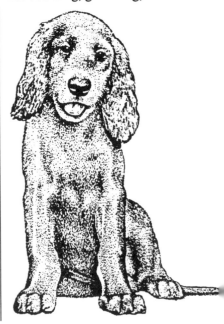

showing your pet. Some facilities will not accept vaccinations done at low-cost clinics, due to the questionable practices at some of these places. This means you'll have to pay for your pet to be revaccinated; while revaccination will not harm your pet, it is an unnecessary expense you can prevent.

Do-It-Yourself Vaccinations. Some pharmacies and pet supply catalogs sell over-the-counter vaccine kits for you to administer the vaccinations yourself. As with low-cost clinics, there are problems with this practice.

1. As mentioned above, vaccinations are required for boarding, grooming, and showing your pet. Most facilities will not accept vaccinations done at home, as there is no proof that the vaccinations were done correctly or even done at all! This means you'll have to pay for your pet to be revaccinated, resulting in an unnecessary expense.

2. Vaccinations require special handling and need constant refrigeration. If you purchase vaccines at a grocery store pharmacy, how do you know they were refrigerated promptly upon arrival and not kept on the hot loading dock all day? Did you promptly refrigerate the vaccines after purchase, or did they spend a few hours on the hot dashboard of your car while you ran other errands?

3. What if you accidentally vaccinate yourself while attempting to vaccinate your dog? This happens frequently; while you won't catch any of the diseases contained within the vaccine, you can develop a nasty infected abscess.

4. What if your puppy jumps at the wrong time and you only get half the vaccine in him, squirting the rest into the air? Should you revaccinate him, or is half a vaccine good enough?

5. Vaccinating at home means your puppy won't receive that very important annual examination and fecal test. While you can bring your puppy to the doctor just for these two things, you won't save any money doing this and may spend even more (most doctors price the vaccinations as a package; if you only need part of the package, such as the exam and fecal test, you still pay full price).

6. What if your pet develops a vaccine reaction after receiving its immunization? Can you get your puppy to the doctor in enough time for proper treatment? While most reactions are

not life-threatening, some are; prompt treatment is needed.

7. While we never expect our own pets to bite us, it can happen. Giving a shot can be painful. What if your dog bites you as a result of the painful injection?

8. You can't legally give a rabies injection; only a licensed veterinarian can do that. This means you will still have to see your doctor for that. Most veterinarians charge a full office call in addition to the rabies injection, meaning you'll save no money asking for just the rabies vaccine.

Your puppy will need a series of vaccinations until it is about 4 months old. The specific vaccinations that are needed are discussed below. These will vary from doctor to doctor; for now, it's important to understand what vaccines do, what they don't do, and why your new puppy needs so many.

2 Months Old (8 Weeks)

First puppy vaccinations (distemper-hepatitis-leptospirosis-parainfluenza-parvo virus-corona virus (DHLPP-C))

WHEN TO VACCINATE FOR LYME'S DISEASE . . . . .

A new disease and new vaccine have prompted a lot of questions from pet owners. Lyme's disease was first reported in people in Lyme County, Connecticut. Since that time, owners have been concerned about their pets contracting this disease and potentially spreading it to people.

Until recently, there was debate about whether or not dogs even got Lyme's disease. While it was known that many dogs tested positive for Lyme's disease on blood tests, these dogs also failed to ever become ill. Some dogs with symptoms suggestive of Lyme's disease (swollen, painful joints, fever) responded to antibiotic therapy despite lack of definitive proof of the disease.

When the vaccine for Lyme's disease was introduced, many doctors advised vaccination for all puppies and adult dogs, even though the chance of exposure to the infectious agent (which is acquired through ticks) was extremely limited.

3 Months Old (12 Weeks)

Second puppy vaccinations
(DHLPP-C, kennel cough)

4 Months Old (16 Weeks)

Third puppy vaccinations
(DHLPP-C, kennel cough, rabies)

What Vaccines Do...

When your puppy receives an
injection, it receives either a
killed bacteria or virus or a
modified live virus. These
bacterium and viruses are killed
or modified in such a way that
they will stimulate the puppy's
immune system to produce
antibodies but not harm the
puppy. Think of a vaccine as a
source of foreign protein. When
this foreign protein, called an
antigen, is introduced into your
puppy's body, the body will
make antibodies against that protein (certain types of white blood
cells will also be stimulated to
provide a so-called "cell-medi-
ated" immunity; however, to
keep things simple, we'll just
concentrate on the antibodies).
These antibodies will protect the
puppy the next time that foreign
protein enters the body, as when
the puppy might be exposed to
the actual disease. These antibodies will protect the puppy from

---

Whether or not you have your puppy vaccinated for this disease depends upon several factors that you should discuss with
your veterinarian:

••➡ Certain areas of the country have a higher incidence of the
disease. If you live in one of these areas it may be advisable to vaccinate against Lyme's disease.

••➡ If you live in an area with a large tick population (such as a
rural area), vaccination may be wise.

••➡ Dogs that spend a lot of time outdoors in areas which are
prone to tick infestations (hunting areas, parks, or wooded areas)
may benefit from the vaccination.

Diagnosis is difficult. When detected and treated early, dogs with
Lyme's disease usually respond quickly and suffer few ill effects.

the disease. An unvaccinated puppy will also make antibodies against the disease, but the disease may kill the puppy before the antibodies have a chance to work. Pets are vaccinated annually to restimulate the body to produce more antibodies, as the antibodies don't last forever.

What Vaccines Don't Do...

No vaccine is perfect. A vaccine depends upon several things in order to work.

The puppy must be capable of mounting an immune response and forming antibodies. While this is not a problem for most puppies, there are several times when a puppy may not be able to make antibodies. If the puppy doesn't make antibodies, the vaccine won't work.

1. A puppy won't make antibodies effectively if it's sick. Therefore, it's critical that a thorough examination be performed prior to vaccinating the puppy. Sick puppies should not be vaccinated.

2. A puppy can't make antibodies if it received antibodies from its mother that have not "worn off" yet. Assuming the

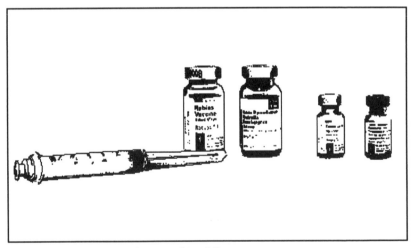

Vacines protect your puppy from a variety of diseases.

mother dog is vaccinated, these "maternal" antibodies pass to the puppy after birth during nursing (specifically in the first one to two days after birth when the puppy consumes the colostrum, or antibody-rich milk). These antibodies offer short-term (usually several weeks to several months) protection against diseases. If a puppy is vaccinated while these maternal antibodies are still present, it will not make any antibodies of its own (see below for further discussion of maternal antibodies and how they affect vaccinations).

3. Rarely, a puppy may be born with a deficient immune system and be incapable of making protective antibodies. These puppies usually die within a few days after birth.

Assuming your puppy is capable of making protective antibodies, vaccinations will stimulate its immune system to make protective antibodies.

Despite what many people think, no vaccine is 100 percent effective. While most puppies that are vaccinated will not contract the disease, there are exceptions.

Here are several things that can happen to a vaccinated puppy that is subsequently exposed to a disease:

•• ➡ Most puppies will not contract the disease at all.

•• ➡ Some puppies will contract the virus or bacterium, shed the virus or bacterium, but never appear ill. Yet, they can pass the virus or bacterium to other puppies.

•• ➡ Some puppies will get a mild form of the disease.

•• ➡ In very rare cases, the puppy will get the full-blown disease.

Ideally, your puppy should recieve all of its vaccinations prior to interacting with other pets. While you can allow a partially vaccinated puppy to interact with other pets, there is a slight risk to this practice as your puppy may not be fully protected against communicable diseases.

Vaccinations are important for all puppies and are an inexpensive way to prevent fatal diseases. Follow your doctor's recommendations for vaccinating your puppy.

Common Owner Concerns

Q: It seems like my puppy needs a lot of shots, and the doctor keeps giving her the same ones over and over. Are these additional vaccinations necessary?

A: Antibodies from the mother, called maternal antibodies, are present in any puppy whose mother was vaccinated prior to the pregnancy and who was able to nurse and receive colostrum.

DON'T DO IT YOURSELF!! . . . .

In an attempt to save a few dollars, a few owners vaccinate their pets themselves. Vaccines are inexpensive and can be purchased from many pharmacies or pet supply catalogs. While this may seem like a great way to save on doctor bills, owners should seriously reconsider vaccinating pets themselves. Consider all that could go wrong with at-home vaccinations:

••➡ The vaccine may not be handled correctly. Did the pharmacy promptly refrigerate the vaccine, or was it left on the loading dock in the hot sun all day? Did you store it promptly and properly after purchase, or did you leave it on your hot car dashboard while you ran a few errands? Improperly storing vaccines can cause them to become inactive and useless.

••➡ The vaccine must be given correctly. The instructions and diagrams that accompany the vaccines are often hard to understand and in some cases inaccurate. Improperly giving a vaccine means the vaccine won't work.

••➡ Even though most owners don't think their pet would ever bite them, getting a shot hurts! You put yourself at risk if the pain from the injection causes your pet to unexpectedly bite you!

••➡ Vaccine manufacturers receive many reports each year from owners who accidentally vaccinate themselves. While you won't catch the disease you're vaccinating for, you can get a nasty, infected wound.

Maternal antibodies don't last forever. For some diseases, maternal antibodies disappear by 8 weeks of age, for others, they may be present up to several months of age. While we know the average life of maternal antibodies, we don't know how long they last in any one individual puppy. We know if we vaccinate a puppy against parvo virus, for example, and maternal antibodies against parvo virus are still present, that vaccine offers no protection (the maternal antibodies "interfere" with

---

• •➡ If the pet jerks while receiving an injection, part of the vaccine might be injected into the air and not the pet. This means the pet must be revaccinated.

• •➡ Most states only allow licensed veterinarians to obtain and give a rabies vaccination. Even if you give the other vaccinations yourself, you must still go to a veterinarian for a rabies vaccination. Many doctors charge a full office call just to give a rabies vaccinations.

• •➡ By not using a veterinarian for all vaccinations, you deprive the pet of a yearly physical examination, heartworm test, and fecal analysis for parasites. *The* most important reason for the yearly visit is not the vaccinations but the examination. After all, how many pets do you know that die of rabies, parvovirus, or distemper infection? Very few. The most common causes of death are organ failure (especially heart, kidney, and liver), cancer, and systemic diseases secondary to periodontal infections. These are all things that can be discovered during the annual physical and in most cases successfully treated.

• •➡ Finally, your pet will probably need to be boarded or hospitalized at some time. Unless you can show proof that a veterinarian has vaccinated the pet, both kennels and veterinary hospitals will require revaccination prior to boarding or hospitalization. This means an extra, unnecessary expense.

In the end, it really isn't worth it to attempt at-home vaccinations. There are other ways to save money on health care (see Chapter 13); don't put yourself and your pet at risk to save a few dollars.

our vaccination). Since we don't know exactly when *your* puppy's maternal antibodies will disappear, we "overvaccinate" to be on the safe side. Too many vaccines will not hurt your puppy; undervaccinating it could be fatal. Therefore, veterinarians have developed vaccine protocols to maximize your puppy's ability to produce antibodies.

We also know that repeated vaccinations produce more antibodies than just one vaccination. Giving your puppy several vaccinations for the same disease allows it to produce the maximum amount of antibodies, thus offering the most protection possible.

Q: My puppy seemed listless the day after she got her shots. Is this going to happen after every visit?

A: Some puppies, usually those of smaller breeds, seem to have more "vaccine reactions" than others. Usually, the reactions are mild and may include listlessness and a decreased appetite. Occasionally, a puppy may vomit or have diarrhea after the vaccination. Rarely, repeated vomiting, diarrhea, difficulty breathing, or hives may be seen. If any of these more severe signs occur, your puppy should receive immediate treatment for this allergic reaction.

A puppy that has a reaction after a vaccination will not necessarily have one every time. As the puppy grows, the incidences of vaccine reactions usually decrease or disappear.

Q: After the vaccination, my puppy had a lump on her hip for about three weeks. What caused this?

A: Vaccines are foreign proteins, or antigens. Since the body recognizes vaccines as antigens, a local inflammatory response occurs. The lump you saw was a result of this local inflammation and is called a sterile abscess. As the inflammation subsides and the foreign protein is absorbed and neutralized, the lump should disappear as the body heals itself. These abscesses usually require no treatment and are not painful to your puppy. If there is any doubt as to whether the lump is from the vaccine, the doctor can aspirate the lump and examine it microscopically to determine the cause.

Chapter 4

The First Doctor Visit

· ·

Ideally, you should have your new puppy examined the day of purchase. If your doctor's office is not open the day you purchase your puppy, at least try to schedule the first visit within 24 to 48 hours. It's critical to make sure your puppy is healthy, especially if the party who sold you the puppy gives you a health warranty good for several days following the purchase.

During the first visit, your puppy will probably need some vaccinations. Which vaccinations your puppy will need depends upon whether or not he has had any previous vaccinations and how old he is when you purchase him. Specific vaccinations are discussed in chapters 3 and 12.

The doctor will do several things on the first visit; depending upon whether any illnesses are detected during the visit and how many questions you have, the first visit will take anywhere from 30 to 60 minutes. During the first visit, the vet will:

••➡ Perform a complete physical examination.

••➡ Do a microscopic analysis of the feces ("stool test") for internal parasites.

••➡ Discuss feeding, training, behavior, spaying or neutering, heartworm disease, and what will occur during subsequent visits.

••➡ Answer any questions you may ask.

The Physical Exam

An important part of the visit is the physical examination. This exam is done to determine if your puppy is healthy enough to receive vaccinations, as well as determine if any illnesses or congenital abnormalities exist. If problems are found during the exam, you may desire to return the puppy to the breeder or pet store for a replacement or payment for medical services as allowed by your contract or warranty.

During the exam, the doctor will:

• • ➡ Examine the ears, checking for any unusual odors or exudate (waxy buildup) that might indicate an infection with ear mites, bacteria, and/or yeasts (Chapter 10).

• • ➡ Examine the eyes. They should be clear; the sclera (white part of the eyes) should be white, not red, and have a few small blood vessels present. There should be no large amounts of

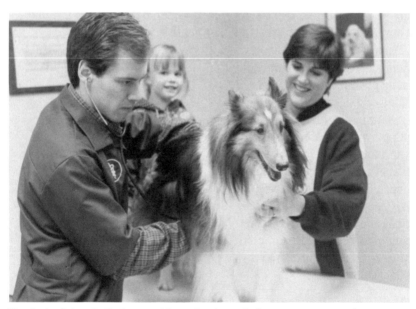

The doctor listens to the heart and lungs for signs of a heart murmer or respiratory infection during the annual physical examination of Tex, a 13-year-old male Shetland sheepdog.

discharge; any drainage that is seen should be clear (some breeds of puppies normally have a small amount of drainage from the eyes).

••➡ Look in the mouth. The doctor wants to be sure the deciduous teeth (baby teeth) are growing in normally, and that the upper and lower teeth touch when the mouth is closed.

Abnormalities of the teeth or jaws may require orthodontic correction. The hard palate is examined to make sure that a cleft palate is not present. The odor of the mouth is noted; foul odors may indicate an oral infection.

••➡ Check the skin and hair coat. There should be no external parasites such as fleas or ticks on

DOES YOUR PET REALLY HAVE A FEVER? . . . .

From time to time you may need to take your puppy's temperature. It's not a difficult procedure, although most owners find it at least a little unpleasant (and puppies find it a bit uncomfortable).

To take your puppy's temperature, purchase a thermometer (preferably one that goes to 106 degrees) and some lubricant (such as K-Y Jelly or even Vasoline). Have someone hold the puppy's head and body, carefully restraining him. Insert the lubricated thermometer about one inch into the puppy's rectum and hold it in place for approximately two minutes. (Have your veterinarian demonstrate this for you before you attempt it for the first time.) When the time is up, remove the thermometer and record the temperature. Be sure to clean the thermometer well and label it for the puppy's use only!

Normal temperature for a puppy is 101.5 (with a range of 100.5-102.5). If the temperature is 103.5 or higher, call your veterinarian. If it is 104 or higher, plan on visiting the doctor.

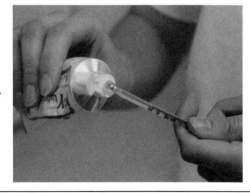

the puppy. No bald spots should be present. The hair should be smooth and shiny, and not rough and unkempt. The skin should be free of lumps, bumps, pimples, and any other skin lesions that might indicate an infection, such as mange or ringworm (Chapter 10).

••➡ Palpate (feel) the abdomen. No pain should be noted during the palpation, nor should any

WORMS ....

Worms are often blamed for many puppy illnesses. While worms can be a problem, other conditions can cause similar diseases.

Worms, more correctly called internal parasites, are often found in the microscopic examination of your puppy's feces. Rarely, worms can actually be seen in the puppy's stool. The most common type of worms that owners actually see in the feces are either roundworms, which look like spaghetti and are only seen in severe infections, or tapeworms, which are flat, resemble grains of rice, and are caused by fleas.

Sometimes, puppies with worms, usually tapeworms, will scoot their rumps on the floor, although scooting is more often seen with anal sac problems.

Regular microscopic examinations of your puppy's feces will help ensure that your puppy stays worm-free. Because so many things can cause diseases in puppies other than internal parasites, owners should refrain from using over-the-counter deworming medications which are often ineffective anyway. Regular use of monthly heartworm preventative medication can help control internal parasites.

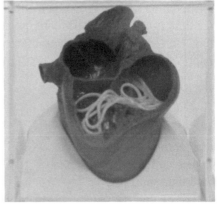

Heartworms are shown in this model of a dog's heart.

KEEPING YOUR PET CLEAN . . . .

New puppy owners often ask how often they can bathe their puppies. While the puppy only needs to be bathed when he gets dirty or smelly (except for those breeds that require regular grooming), most puppies can be bathed regularly. Most veterinarians generally suggest no more than weekly bathing unless the puppy has a skin problem requiring more frequent bathing.

A popular shampoo is HyLyt shampoo, available from your veterinarian. This shampoo is mild, hypoallergenic, soap-free, and contains moisturizers. All of this means that regular bathing won't dry out your puppy's delicate skin like harsher shampoos can. And remember not to use people shampoo unless it's an emergency and your veterinarian okays it. Human products are formulated for human skin, which is structurally different from puppy skin.

Start bathing your puppy when he is young (6-8 weeks) so he will become used to the bathing procedure. Try to make it as pleasant an experience as possible. A tub or a sink works fine: massage water into the coat, use the shampoo, and thoroughly rinse him. If shampoo gets in the puppy's eyes, thoroughly flush them out with water. Drying with a towel or blow dryer is fine. Puppies will not chill and get sick after bathing, so don't be concerned about that.

---

organs feel enlarged. The umbilical (belly-button) area is examined for the presence of a hernia (Chapter 11) that may need surgical correction.

••➡ Listen to the heart and lungs. Occasionally a heart murmur is present, or the heart can't be heard normally on one side of the chest. A murmur is caused by turbulent blood flow in the heart or blood vessels leading from the heart. Heart murmurs in puppies can be innocent (also called physiologic) murmurs or pathologic murmurs. Innocent murmurs (Chapter 11) are soft murmurs that normally disappear by 6 months of age and will not cause the puppy any problem. Pathologic murmurs can be caused by fever, anemia, or problems with the heart valves or blood vessels leading from the heart.

•••➡ Examine the genital system. While most male puppies will have both of their testes in the scrotum by the first visit, some do not. These will often descend by the last visit; if they do not, surgery is needed to neuter the pet and correct the cryptorchid condition (Chapter 11).

Microscopic Fecal Examination

A fresh (less than 24 hours old) sample of your puppy's feces will be examined microscopically for the presence of intestinal parasites (worms). You should plan on bringing a fecal sample to the veterinarian; although he can often obtain one from your puppy, the procedure is a bit uncomfortable (similar to taking its temperature). The feces should be fresh; it's advised to collect it the day before your actual appointment (if you wait until the day of the appointment, the puppy may not eliminate and then you won't have a sample! If you already have a sample and the puppy provides you with a fresh one right before your visit, you can always dispose of the older sample and bring the fresh one). Only a

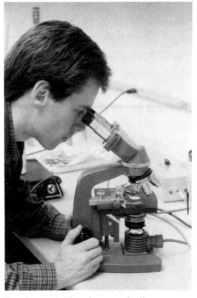

Fecal material is microscopically examined for worms and other parasites.

small sample is needed, roughly one-half teaspoonful. Some owners get a bit overzealous and bring in quite a lot of feces. This is one case where more is definitely *not* better!

The doctor will mix the feces with a sodium nitrate solution that will cause any parasite eggs present to float to the top of the vial, where they are trapped on a glass slide. The slide is then examined microscopically for the eggs.

Alternatively, if a very small sample of feces is available, the doctor may perform a direct

OTC MEDICATIONS. . . . .

In an attempt to save money on veterinary visits, many owners play doctor at home and give their puppies human medications. While many human drugs are used in puppies, this practice should only be done under veterinary supervision. Many human products are not safe for use in pets. Also, pets require different doses than people. Commonly used over-the-counter medications include:

••➡ Aspirin. Aspirin can be used in dogs for mild arthritic pain at low doses. Higher doses can cause gastrointestinal ulcers. Buffered aspirin may be easier on your pet's stomach.

••➡ Non-steroidals. Non-steroidal medications, such as ibuprofen, Advil, or Naprosyn are commonly taken by people for headaches, menstrual cramps, arthritis, and any type of musculoskeletal pain. These drugs are extremely dangerous in dogs; many dogs have been poisoned and killed by well-intentioned owners who treated their pets with their own medicines. These drugs should not be used in dogs; veterinarians rarely prescribe them, and only if other drugs are ineffective and the pet is closely monitored.

••➡ Tylenol. Another drug which kills pets, Tylenol is often used by owners who suspect that their pet has a fever. Fevers are the body's way of protecting itself and should only be controlled if excessively high with medication prescribed by your doctor.

••➡ Antidiarrheals. Pepto Bismol and Kaopectate can be used safely in most puppies if directed by your veterinarian. However, they are generally ineffective for most causes of diarrhea and can be messy to administer. Until your veterinarian has determined the cause of the diarrhea, it's best not to treat the puppy with home remedies.

••➡ Cough medications. While some doctors okay using human cough syrups at home, coughing in puppies is usually associated with kennel cough or internal parasites; cough medicines are likely to be ineffective in these instances.

Always check with your veterinarian before treating your pet at home. While many over-the-counter medications can be used safely, your doctor needs to be aware of any signs of illness in your puppy.

smear of the feces on a micro-
scope slide mixed with a drop of
water. This test is not as accurate
as the flotation but can often detect any eggs that are present. If
your puppy has had diarrhea, the
doctor may do a floatation and a
smear to increase the chances of
finding the eggs.

Owners are often surprised
that a doctor may want to run
more than one fecal sample.
Many doctors check the feces at
each puppy visit, some check it
just once, and some check a sample on the first and last puppy
visit. Worms are not continu-
ously laying eggs; it may be that
your puppy has worms but they

were not laying eggs the particular day that the feces were
checked. Failure to check the
feces again could mean that your
puppy has worms but they were
missed due to the one negative
sample.

Discussion of Puppy Information

Unless you have other dogs, you
probably don't know much about
your new puppy. While books,
breeders, pet store employees,
and well-intentioned friends may
feel they know it all, your veterinarian has received years of
training in school and post doc-

STEROIDS . . . .

A class of drugs commonly used by veterinarians is the corticosteroids. These drugs are used for many conditions, including
reducing inflammation, relieving the pain of arthritis, treating
animals in shock, treating cancers and autoimmune diseases, and
relieving the itchiness associated with many types of allergic diseases. These are not the same class of steroids that is discussed in
the media, namely the anabolic steroids taken by athletes for
improved performance.

While corticosteroids are truly wonder drugs that can relieve
many problems in dogs, they have disadvantages. Common short-
term side effects include increased appetite, increased thirst, and
increased urination (from the increased water intake). Rarely,
some dogs will act "spaced out," hyperexcitable, or even lethargic

toral continuing education in his field. He is uniquely qualified to instruct you on the proper care of your new puppy. Take the advice from others with a grain of salt; these well-intentioned friends might think they know it all, but they have not received formal training in veterinary medicine. Follow your doctor's advice when it comes to caring for your new family member!

Several areas of concern should be discussed during the visit. These concerns include housetraining, biting, barking, general puppy behavior problems, spaying or neutering versus breeding, a lifeplan for your puppy, an explanation of what vaccinations need to be given and when, heartworm disease and prevention, bathing, brushing the puppy's teeth, grooming needs, including home care of nails and coat, feeding, vitamins, parasite control (if needed), and any other concerns that may affect your puppy (such as hip dysplasia for large breed puppies).

Ask Questions

You are paying for the doctor's time, so make the most of your visit. Bring a list of questions for the doctor. No question is stupid! Even though the doctor may

---

or drunk. These side effects wear off shortly after the medication is stopped.

Long-term side effects from chronic use include osteoporosis, liver disease, diabetes, decreased wound healing, increased susceptibility to infections, Cushing's disease (a condition of too much steroid in the body) and Addison's disease (a shock-like condition that occurs if steroids, which have been used chronically, are suddenly stopped).

Long-term side effects can be prevented by treating the pet with other medications if they are available, such as antihistamines in allergic conditions. In cases where corticosteroids need to be used for a long period of time (cancers, autoimmune diseases like lupus), the pet is carefully monitored and the lowest effective dose possible is used. If your veterinarian prescribes "steriods" for your pet, be sure to discuss the pros and cons and side effects of the medication.

GIVING YOUR PUPPY MEDICINE . . . .

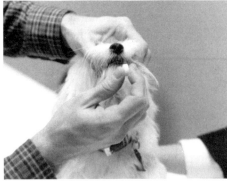

Giving your puppy a tablet.

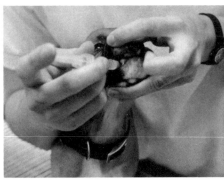

Liquid medicines are easily administered with a syringe.

have heard the question before, YOU have never asked it before, and you deserve an answer. If your doctor rushes you or refuses to answer questions, it's time to look for another doctor!

Common Owner Concerns

Q: The breeder has already given my puppy her first set of shots, yet the doctor wants to revaccinate her. Is there a need for this extra expense?

A: Some doctors feel the need to revaccinate puppies that have already had some vaccinations. It may be that your doctor doesn't trust the particular breeder who sold you your puppy. Maybe he feels that breeder used the incorrect vaccine, or that it was given at too early an age. If you trust your doctor, rest assured that he isn't revaccinating your new puppy just to make a few extra dollars. If you are uncomfortable and don't trust him, you may want to consider looking for another veterinarian for your pet. Remember, though, that the doctor does know more about health care than any breeder, so I would tend to believe him over a breeder or other pet supplier.

Q: Is it really necessary that our puppy have an examination on every visit? She seems healthy and the examinations are just another expense. This puppy is costing us a lot of money!

A: You are beginning to realize just how expensive owning a puppy actually can be for its owner. Hopefully, all potential puppy owners will do their homework *before* purchasing their pet and make sure they can afford the care required by this new family member.

A complete physical examination is critical on each and every visit. Your puppy is rapidly growing and changing. Problems not present on the previous examinations may become apparent on future visits. Realize that the most important part of every veterinary visit is the examination and not the vaccinations. Take advantage of each visit to discuss any questions or concerns you have about your puppy's health or behavior.

Chapter 5
Feeding Your Puppy

· ·

Three of the most common questions new puppy owners ask are "What do I feed my puppy," "How often do I feed him," and "How much do I feed him?" The simple and correct answers are, respectively, "Premium puppy food," "Feed as often as he gets hungry," and "Feed him as much as he needs to eat"! Unfortunately, these answers don't offer a lot of help to new owners. In order to answer these questions, it's first necessary to understand something about pet food. While you don't need a Ph.D. in nutrition to properly feed your puppy, it does make sense to have a basic understanding of nutrition to ensure that your puppy will get everything it needs.

Nutrients

Your puppy needs many nutrients to not only sustain life but to encourage growth, promote a healthy coat, and allow proper function of its organs and immune system. An improperly nourished puppy is unhealthy and is prone to illness. Preventing illness with proper nutrition is an important part of a pet owner's responsibility.

Water While most people forget about water as a nutrient, it is without a doubt the most important one. An animal can survive after losing most of its fat or protein, but a 15 percent loss of body water results in death! Your puppy's body, just like your body, is made up mostly of water. While food can supply a little or a lot of the puppy's daily water needs, your pet should always have a fresh bowl of clean water. An exception might be made when housebreaking your new puppy—you may decide to remove water from its cage at night. That's fine, as long as water was available throughout the day and will be offered in the morning.

Dry food is 6 to 10 percent water, soft-moist is 23 to 40 percent water, and canned food is 68 to 78 percent water. As a rule, the amount of water consumed by mature dogs is about 2.5 times the amount of dry matter consumed in food.

Water should be increased in times of illness, when fever is present, when the temperature increases, if your puppy pants excessively, or if certain medications (such as corticosteroids) are given which result in an increased urinary output.

Energy For simplicity's sake, energy is provided in food by fats, carbohydrates, and proteins. The energy content of food is defined in kilocalories, which is 1,000 calories (in nutrition language, the word calorie usually means kilocalorie). If the food is a premium food and correctly balanced, as a rule feeding the amount needed to meet the puppy's energy requirement provides the proper amount of all its needed nutrients. The amount to feed can be calculated by dividing the animal's energy requirement by the energy density of the food. In practice, most owners don't wish to do this. Pet food companies have already done this and offer a suggested amount to feed on the food package; the amount varies with the pet's weight.

Carbohydrates Carbohydrates are composed of sugars, starches, and fiber. Carbohydrates are excellent sources of energy in puppy foods. Excess carbohydrates in the diet that are not needed by the puppy are stored as body fat.

Fiber is used to add bulk to the diet to prevent both diarrhea and constipation. Fiber also helps the animal feel full so it doesn't become obese. Cheaper pet foods often have too much fiber; puppies become full before consuming the needed nutrients and can exhibit nutritional deficiencies.

Protein Protein is composed of amino acids, which are the "building blocks" of the body.

Proteins are used as enzymes, hormones, and in making muscle and other structural tissues. While people often mistakenly are concerned about the protein content of food, in reality it's the amino acids that are important. The protein sources used in formulating the diet must contain the proper amounts of the essential amino acids needed by the pet, or it will suffer from an amino acid deficiency despite an adequate protein intake. Excess dietary protein can increase the stress on the pet's kidneys and may cause harm in the long run.

Fat Fats are used for energy as well as being needed for the absorption of vitamins A, D, E, and K. Fats also are used in the body's productions of hormones. Fats also make diets more palatable. Excess concentrations of fats can lead to obesity, hepatic lipidosis (fatty liver disease), and pancreatitis.

Fat deficiency, or rather fatty acid deficiency, is rare in pets. Certain fatty acids can be supplemented by your doctor to help with certain skin problems, specifically atopic dermatitis, a form of allergic dermatitis.

Minerals Minerals include such things as calcium, phospho-

rus, iron, and zinc, among others. As a rule, minerals function as co-enzymes which help control numerous biochemical reactions in the body. Minerals also are constituents of bone and muscle. Mineral deficiencies rarely occur in pets, with the exception of zinc deficiency (see below). Mineral excess can occur by overzealous administration of minerals by owners, specifically calcium and phosphorus. Many owners give their growing puppies calcium pills, thinking it will help with skeletal growth. Too much calcium can actually cause problems. Mineral supplementation is not recommended unless directed by your veterinarian.

Zinc deficiency can result from excess dietary calcium (seen when owners supplement puppy food with calcium pills) or in cheap, generic pet foods. Many cheap pet foods are deficient in zinc; puppies that eat this diet usually show signs of zinc deficiency, which include crusty, scaly skin. In people, a similar condition is called acrodermatitis enteropathica. The disease in puppies often occurs with cheap, generic foods that contain excess calcium, phytic acid (common in plant proteins which make up a large part of generic diets), copper, and cadmium. These substances bind the zinc in the diet, reducing its absorption by the intestines. The disease may only be seen in puppies eating certain lots of generic foods, as generic foods vary in their nutritional content from lot to lot (another reason generic foods are very inexpensive and inadequate nutritionally for your puppy). Treatment involves zinc supplementation and switching to a premium diet.

Vitamins Like minerals, vitamins function as enzymes or co-enzymes. Pure vitamin deficiencies or toxicities are rarely encountered in puppies, as pet food manufacturers "overcompensate" and make sure the food contains more than enough of these compounds. There are a few rare exceptions: Vitamin A toxicity can result during the course of treating a certain type of skin disease, vitamin A deficiency seborrhea. This disease is rare and usually would occur in an older dog. Owners treating this condition under a doctor's guidance are warned about the signs of vitamin A toxicity so treatment can be altered at the first signs of problems.

Vitamin K deficiency can rarely occur as a result of chronic diarrhea, acute poisoning by warfarin-type rat poisons, if poor-quality diets are fed which contain an insufficient amount of fat, and as a result of certain antibiotic therapy.

Thiamin deficiency can result in pets fed exclusively fish diets; since fish is not a normal food for dogs, this would not be expected in most puppies but is seen in cats.

Large amounts of ingested raw egg whites can result in a biotin deficiency; however, this is also rare.

Which Brand Of Food?

Now that you have a basic understanding of nutrition, the next step is to understand the differences in pet foods. Some seem to cost a lot, whereas others are extremely inexpensive. With so many choices, how do you know what food is right for your puppy? Can reading the labels help, or are they another source of confusion?

While breeders, groomers, and clerks at the pet stores all have their own opinions about the "best" brand of food, realize that once again your doctor has been trained in nutrition. He is the best source to turn to for nutritional advice.

However, doctors can also be biased. Due to intense competition from the large number of veterinarians, doctors feel pressure to sell pet food in their offices as well. You could easily assume that your doctor is biased toward the brand he sells. While there may be some truth to that, your doctor has a variety of brands he could choose to sell. Most doctors do their homework and select one to several brands they feel are the best.

In deciding what food is best for your puppy, realize that all puppies are different. What is

YOU CAN'T JUDGE A LABEL BY WHAT IT SAYS . . . .

Many clients say that they feed a particular brand of pet food based on the advice of a breeder, groomer, or pet store clerk. While these sources are well intentioned and may have a favorite brand, they are not doctors. Veterinarians receive formal training in nutrition and diseases that can result from improper nutrition. Take your veterinarian's advice on the proper food for your pet. Puppies require one type of food, adult animals another, and geriatric pets still another.

Be careful what the label says too. Many clients tell me that the label on their brand of food claims it is nutritionally complete and therefore are convinced it must be a good food. Here are a few tips on reading the pet food labels.

1. *Guaranteed Analysis.* This states the minimum levels of nutrients in the food. A food with a minimum level of 5 percent protein means that the food has at least 5 percent protein; it may have a lot more, possibly even too much! Also, there is no guarantee that this protein is a good-quality protein. Chicken feathers have at least 5 percent protein, but I promise you that your pet won't get any nutrients from this protein source!

2. *Digestibility.* Poultry meal is a common protein source, but the digestibility of protein meals varies from poor to excellent.

best for your puppy may not be best for your neighbor's puppy. The neighbor's pet may not find your puppy's food palatable, maybe your puppy's food even makes the neighbor's pet sick. Obviously, consulting with a doctor to find the right choice of food makes sense.

Grocery Store, Pet Store, Discount Store, or Doctor's Office? There are several classifications of foods available for your puppy. Generic or private-label foods are the least expensive but also least healthy for your pet. Owners should avoid this type of food, as health

Reputable manufacturers use higher-quality ingredients; the quality of the ingredient is reflected in the cost of the food. Stay away from poorly digestible, cheaper generic brands.

3. *Nutritional Adequacy.* Many products state that the food has been "formulated to meet the nutrition levels established by the AAFCO." Unfortunately, this just guarantees the food meets a mathematical minimum number. Your pet may not be able to digest or absorb anything in it, because the food never had to go through feeding trials to assess palatability, digestibility, and nutrition merit.

"Animal feeding tests using AAFCO procedures that substantiate that this food provides complete and balanced nutrition" means the food has been fed to many pets for extended periods of time and that no nutritional problems were detected. The better, more expensive brands use this designation after conducting costly feeding trials.

4. *Cost.* There's nothing wrong with trying to save a buck *if* you're not putting your pet's health at risk. A recent survey of pet foods showed that a premium brand costs no more than the average cost of the nine most popular grocery store brands.

Unfortunately, you can't rely on the label to differentiate between pet foods. Your veterinarian has been trained in nutrition. Follow his advice when determining the proper food for your pets. Usually, the cost of the diets at his office are very competitive with pet stores and in some cases even cheaper.

problems such as zinc or fatty acid deficiency may result.

Grocery stores carry popular brands of food, such as those made by Gaines, Purina, and Kennel Ration, among others. Most of these foods have been around for years, have undergone extensive research and feeding trials, and are acceptable choices of foods for your puppy.

Premium foods are available at many pet stores and veterinary hospitals. They have the highest-quality ingredients available in pet foods; as a result of the high-quality ingredients, they tend to be the most expensive.

Obviously, there are many sources competing for your pet food dollar. Choosing a pet food is important and should not be done hastily. It would even be wise to discuss the choice with your veterinarian *before* you purchase your puppy. Having to buy food on the spur of the moment after purchasing the puppy is not a good idea.

The price of pet foods is determined by many things. These include marketing and advertising, feeding trials, and quality of ingredients. The *cost* of pet foods, which is different from the *price* of the foods, is exactly how much it costs to feed the pet at each meal. The cost of the food is really more important than the price. For example, a generic brand of food has a lower price than a premium brand, but actually costs more. Why? Let's suppose that due to the high bulk content of the generic food, a 10-pound bag lasts only two weeks for your pet because he has to eat so much of it to get his required daily energy. Let's suppose that same 10-pound bag of premium food lasts eight weeks; because of the high-quality ingredients, the pet doesn't need to eat as much. The price of the premium food may be more for each bag, but because it lasts longer the cost is lower. With the premium food, there will probably be less feces produced each day (a desirable quality for pet owners). Feeding premium food may result in fewer doctor bills since the food is a better diet for the pet. While the cost of the ingredients in premium diets is higher than in generic diets, the health benefits and the smaller amount of food needed at each feeding compensate for the higher-priced ingredients.

There is some concern about whether these premium foods actually result in better health than the popular grocery store brands. There is no current research to show the extra benefit when compared to popular store brands that have undergone similar testing (feeding trials). However, due to intense competition the price difference between premium brands and popular brands is fairly small.

In helping you and your doctor decide whether a premium brand or popular brand should be offered, consider that the main difference is quality of ingredients. A typical premium brand might have whole dressed chicken as a main ingredient, whereas the popular brand might contain chicken parts or by-products. While chicken by-products are not bad, the nutritional value is not quite as good as whole chicken.

These are just some of the factors to consider when deciding if a premium food is best for your puppy or if you would prefer a popular store brand. There are other factors to consider when selecting a food, however.

Palatability   No matter how good the nutrients are in a particular puppy food, he must eat it! While that may sound obvious, not every puppy likes every food. Palatability is a measure of how palatable or tasty a particular food is. Several factors

influence the palatability of a food:

••➡ Food temperature—Food warmed to body temperature is more palatable than food at room temperature; warming the food is often advised for puppies that don't seem interested in a food or when the puppy is ill. Warming only works for canned food; warm water can be added to dry food for a similar effect.

••➡ Odor—Dogs have an excellent sense of smell so the food must smell good for the pet to eat it. Warming increases odor; pets with blocked nasal passages (from illness) may not be able to smell the food and may not eat it.

••➡ Texture—Some pets prefer a certain feel or shape of food; because of its texture, canned food is always preferred over dry food.

••➡ Nutrient content—Foods with a higher fat content are preferred over food that are high in fiber, so-called diet foods.

••➡ Habit—Most pets prefer the diet to which they are accustomed; new foods should be introduced slowly.

Acceptability   Just because a food is palatable doesn't mean your puppy will accept it. In order for food to be accepted, the puppy must obviously be hungry and have a need for the food. Additionally, the puppy must not show an aversion to the food. If the food previously made the puppy sick, he may not want to eat it.

Optimum Nutrient Content
Foods available for sale must list on the bag that the food met guidelines established by the AAFCO (Association of American Feed Control Officials). The AAFCO statement will either say that the diet has been "formulated to meet the nutrition levels established by the AAFCO" or "animal feeding tests using AAFCO procedures substantiate that this food pro-

vides complete and balanced nutrition."

Unfortunately, food that just meets nutrition levels may not be adequate for your puppy. This designation just guarantees the food meets a mathematical minimum. Your pet may not be able to digest or absorb anything in it, because the food never had to go through feeding trials to assess palatability and digestibility or show if the animals in the trials grew or suffered malnutrition.

Diets that have gone through extensive feeding trials often cost more than generic foods but are preferred. Food that has been tested through feeding trials has been fed to many pets for

---

CHANGING FOODS . . . .

You rarely have to offer your puppy a different brand of food, but there's nothing wrong with doing so if you want to offer the puppy variety. However, there is a secret to switching brands of food. Switching to a new brand overnight may cause vomiting or diarrhea in a few dogs; some pets are finicky and may not eat a new diet that is suddenly introduced.

The best way to offer your pet a new diet is by gradually introducing it. When you have about a week's worth of the old diet remaining, purchase the new food. Add about 10 percent of the new diet each day, gradually adding more until you run out of the old food and the pet is eating only the new diet. This trick usually prevents upset tummies and eases the transition to the new food.

extended periods of time with no nutritional problem detected.

Supplementation Premium diets are complete and balanced and do not need to be supplemented with "people food." While some pets suffer no ill effects from eating small amounts of certain people foods, other pets don't do as well. Many pets can develop diarrhea or vomit after eating food other than their own. Some pets can develop pancreatitis, an often fatal disease than can be brought on by eating foods high in fat content. Also, some human foods can be toxic, such as chocolate, or hard for the pet to digest, such as milk. Unless your doctor advises otherwise, avoid giving your puppy people food and offer it only premium-quality puppy food.

Prozyme Prozyme is an enzyme supplement that contains cellulase, among other enzymes. Cellulase breaks down cellulose, a constituent of plant cell walls. Since plant material can be found as a component in all pet foods, it is theorized that prozyme might make some nutrients available to the puppy by breaking down these cell walls. Many doctors recommend Prozyme as a way to increase the digestion and absorption of nutrients in the pet's food. Keep in mind that no nutritional supplement will improve a poor-quality diet. As with any nutritional supplement, Prozyme should not be given to your pet without discussing it with your veterinarian.

Additives Some pet owners who fear additives look for additive-free food. Recent research, however, confirms what doctors have said all along: additives rarely cause any problem—they account for 5 percent or less of food-sensitivity problems in pets.

Obesity

While obesity is extremely rare in puppies less than one year old, it is something that can occur or be prevented as a result of feeding habits and behavioral patterns established during puppyhood.

Surprisingly, obesity is the most common nutritional disease in pets, as in people. It is estimated that up to 45 percent of dogs are affected. It seems to occur in neutered dogs more than in intact dogs, especially in spayed females. Certain breeds seem more likely to become obese, including Labrador retrievers, cocker spaniels,

HOW MANY CALORIES ARE IN THOSE PUPPY TREATS? . . . .

Next time you reach for that puppy treat, you may want to stop and consider how many calories are in it. Many owners are amazed that a small puppy that gets just "a few treats a day" doesn't seem to have much of an appetite. When you consider that even a few treats can supply most of a puppy's daily calories, it's real easy to ruin an appetite.

	Calories		Calories
Small dog biscuit	20	1 oz. cheese	106
Medium biscuit	40	1 cookie	140
Large biscuit	120	1 oz. cracker	130
"Lite" biscuit	13	1/4 cup ice cream	66
1 slice of bacon	46	2 oz. hot dog	170
1 oz. candy	130	1 egg	80

dachshunds, beagles, collies, Shetland sheepdogs, basset hounds, and Cairn terriers.

Obesity is usually defined as a body weight of 15 percent above the ideal body weight. While that doesn't seem like a lot, consider that a dog whose ideal body weight should be 10 pounds would be obese if he weighed just 11.5 pounds! Owners who feel that their dogs weigh just a little too much don't realize that for some dogs, weighing a little too much could equate with being dangerously obese.

You can easily feel the ribs of a normal dog who has just a small amount of body fat. Difficulty in feeling the ribs indicates obesity. If you are unable to feel your pet's ribs, it is dangerously obese.

Diets high in fat or sugar are more likely to result in obesity. Obesity results when the excess energy in the diet is stored by an increase in either the number or size of the fat cells. Since the number of fat cells can increase primarily during pregnancy through six months of life, over-feeding puppies increases their fat cell numbers, which makes them prone to obesity later in life. It is recommended to avoid overfeeding; a slightly thin puppy is preferable to an over weight puppy.

In obese pets, the overall energy expenditure is decreased; some obese pets maintain obesity on a diet which contains fewer calories than the diet of their normal weight counterparts. In essence, their body weight set-points are lowered as a result of obesity. This is the reason that obese pets have a lot of trouble losing weight even on store-bought "lite" diets and must be placed on a medically supervised diet that is severely restricted in calories.

Obesity can also be caused by certain hormonal conditions in dogs. Some of the hormonal problems that should be investigated as a cause of obesity include low thyroid levels (hypothyroidism), high cortisol levels (seen in a disease called hyperadrenocorticism, which usually results from a tumor or enlargement of the adrenal glands), pancreatic tumors, or low sex hormones after neutering or spaying. It should be pointed out that neutering and spaying per se do not result in weight gain. Rather, the removal of the sex hormones may be associated with a

decreased energy expenditure. Failing to decrease food intake after neutering or spaying may result in obesity.

Complications of obesity can include diabetes, hypertension (a disease that is only now being recognized frequently in dogs), liver disease, abnormal drug metabolism (which can result in toxic levels of normally "safe" medications as well as prolonged recovery from anesthesia), cardiovascular disease, decreased respiratory capacity (which can increase the risk of anesthesia and strenuous exercise), bone and joint problems (arthritis), cancer, reduced resistance to disease, and dermatitis.

Controlling obesity and preventing its recurrence involve feeding a diet severely restricted in energy under the supervision of your veterinarian. Moderately increase exercise and alter your owner/pet behavior (eliminate begging and the need for treats, don't feed your pet at the table, etc.). Starvation, feeding your pet "a little less," is not recommended; this practice is dangerous and usually results in a decreased ratio of muscle tissue to fat. Using store-bought "lite" diets usually fails to reduce the weight but may, in a few selected instances, help

---

LAMB AND RICE ...
NOT ALWAYS THE BEST CHOICE ....

Recently, many pet owners have jumped on the "lamb and rice" bandwagon. Pet food manufacturers, in their attempts to sell yet another type of food, have pushed lamb and rice diets as the newest, best things for pets. A big selling point is that these diets are "hypoallergenic"; by feeding them, your pet should never have food allergies.

   While there is nothing inherently wrong with lamb and rice diets, there are some things to consider before spending extra money on this special diet:

•• ➡ Food allergies are extremely rare in pets; less than 10 percent of puppies and dogs will ever develop a food allergy.

---

maintain the reduced weight once the ideal weight has been reached. Exercise without calorie restriction is not effective in yielding significant weight loss.

Common Owner Concerns
• •

Q: Does my puppy really need vitamins?

A: Assuming your puppy is eating a high-quality diet, which contains ample vitamins and minerals, he does not need additional vitamins. As with people, however, administering one or two puppy vitamin tablets each day will not harm the pet (as long as your doctor okays it). While he does not *need* the vita-mins, puppies also do not *need* treats, yet most owners give their puppies all sorts of treats. Since one or two puppy vitamins a day won't hurt the puppy, offering him this low-fat, low-salt alternative to store-bought treats will ensure that he receives all the vitamins and minerals he needs (especially if his food intake is down a bit because of hot weather or a minor illness), and is an excellent way to reinforce

••➡ There is nothing inherently hypoallergenic about lamb or rice. Food allergies are more likely to be caused by a protein source that the pet has been eating for some time, often several years.

••➡ Pets diagnosed with food allergies need a hypoallergenic diet. If your pet is used to eating lamb, it will be difficult and expensive to find a suitable diet. Other diet choices for pets with food allergies include fish, turkey, shrimp, lobster, or venison.

••➡ Many lamb and rice diets also contain egg, wheat, soy, beef, and chicken. Your puppy could develop allergies to any or all of these substances despite eating a "lamb and rice" diet.

Since your puppy doesn't derive any extra nutritional benefit from lamb, save your money and feed him a diet recommended by your doctor. If he is ever diagnosed with a food allergy, then your veterinarian may recommend a lamb-based diet as a treatment.

the puppy-owner bond that is so critical to establish between owners and pets. It's probably wise to offer him a vitamin or two each day.

Q: Is one brand of food any better than another? It seems like there are so many brands available at the pet store.

A: As a rule, if you buy a premium brand then all are about equal in quality. Even many store-bought brands are fine-quality products. As long as you avoid generic brands, feeding any brand of high-quality food should ensure proper nutrition for your puppy. Make sure your puppy is fed a diet that is spe-cially formulated for puppies and not adult dogs. Read the label to make sure the food was tested in AAFCO feeding trials. Since there are so many brands available, it is wise to consult with your puppy's veterinarian for advice. He is trained in nutrition; the part-time pet store employees don't have the knowledge of your pet or the training to make nutritional recommendations.

Q: Occasionally my puppy doesn't eat everything we offer her. Should I be concerned?

A: Puppies, like people, occasionally skip a meal or don't eat everything you offer. Assuming the puppy is not acting sick, there is no cause for alarm. Your puppy knows when it is hungry. Various things, including the amount of food in its stomach, feeding-related hormones, blood sugar and fat levels, and even the weather (dogs seem to eat less in the summer heat) all determine how much your pet will eat at any given time.

Q: My veterinarian recommends dry food, yet our puppy really enjoys the canned variety. Is one form better than the next?

A: Pet food can either be dry, semimoist, or canned. Semimoist or dry food are often recommended as they cost considerably less than canned (where you pay for the can and a large amount of water) or semimoist. While canned food does taste better and is therefore preferred by puppies, dry food may help control periodontal disease by reducing tartar build-up.

Q: My puppy doesn't eat his meals regularly. He seems to be picky, eating a lot at one meal and then refusing food at the next. Should I be concerned about this? I hope he's getting enough to eat.

A: Like some children, some puppies can be picky eaters. While most puppies eat everything in sight and still seem to be hungry, there are other puppies that are picky and almost "cat-like" in their appetites. Assuming your puppy is acting normally otherwise and is healthy, he will eat whatever his body needs to sustain itself (and even grow as well). Rest assured that not all puppies that are picky eaters will remain that way as adult dogs. Even if yours does, as long as he seems healthy and is maintaining his weight there is no cause for concern. Your puppy's body will tell him when he needs to eat.

Chapter 6
Socializing Your New Puppy

· ·

Correctly socializing your puppy is the most important thing you can do to prevent future behavioral problems. The most common reason for euthanasia is a behavioral problem; therefore, preventing behavioral problems is critical to decreasing the number of unwanted pets.

The socialization period (3-12 weeks of age) is the period of time early in your puppy's life when it learns to get along with other beings, including people, other species of pets, and other dogs. This period is basically the time when your puppy learns that he is a puppy. The socialization period is a critical time in your puppy's life. He's going through a lot of learning, trying to adjust to his new home and to all the things out in the world.

This period is a time of trying new things, exploring the environment, learning what's safe and what's dangerous, learning the difference between good and bad behaviors, and understanding the difference between punishment and reward.

Any interactions the puppy has during this time have a profound and lasting effect on him. It is critical to maximize good experiences and minimize bad experiences. Now is the time to set boundaries, teaching the puppy what behavior is acceptable and what behavior is unacceptable.

At 5-7 weeks, the puppy approaches any warm body without fear. This is the ideal time for learning to begin, for the puppy to be exposed to as many types

CRYING IN THE NIGHT........................

Occasionally a young puppy, usually 5-12 weeks old, that is placed in a new home goes through a short period of adjustment. Often the puppy has been living with littermates and his mother and is now taken away from this safe environment, placed into a new, strange home, and is left alone at night with no warm body for comfort or snuggling. This is traumatic for the puppy and this separation anxiety is often manifested by crying the first few nights in the new home.

The worst thing you can do is to get up every time the puppy whines. Taking the puppy to bed with you or placing it in your room is even worse. Doing this will develop a habit that is hard to

of people (short, tall, thin, fat, old, young, black, white, etc.) as possible.

The eighth week of age marks the start of stable learning. This is a great time to begin housetraining your puppy. Try to maximize positive experiences; any traumatic experience that occurs starting from the eighth week of life until approximately the twelfth week can permanently affect your puppy.

By 12 weeks of age, the puppy starts to avoid interaction with species (including types of people) it hasn't had contact with during its socialization period. Positive behavior should be reinforced again at this age. If the puppy hasn't had contact with a variety of people and animals, now is the time (and possibly the

last time) you can attempt socialization of these species with your new puppy. Keep in mind that your puppy will not be fully immunized at this age and there is a very slight risk of contracting disease. Make sure any other animals he comes in contact with are currently vaccinated.

While the 8- to 12-week period is critical in socializing your puppy, it will no doubt have some negative experiences during this time. Several of these experiences occur at the veterinarian's office. During these 8-12 weeks of age, the puppy will make two or more visits to the doctor. These visits can be traumatic and even painful due to the necessity for vaccinations. Your doctor should try and make the experience as comfortable break as the puppy learns that whenever he whines, you respond. To speed up the socialization process, it's best to leave the puppy alone. It's certainly okay to check on it when it starts whining and even take the puppy outside in case the whining signals the need to eliminate. If it doesn't eliminate after 10-15 minutes, just place the puppy back in the cage, say a few soothing words, pat it gently on the head, and go back to bed. If your puppy does eliminate outside, make sure to praise it for alerting you to this fact and be happy that your puppy is learning housetraining so easily.

Like parents with a new baby, new puppy owners should plan on missing some sleep the first week or so. Leaving the radio on or placing a blanket or hot water bottle in the cage may help but are not cure-alls.

and pleasant as possible. Praising and rewarding the puppy for good behavior at the veterinary visits can help as well. Remember that puppies can sense and react to the emotions of their owners. If you are uncomfortable at the visit, your puppy will be as well. Don't overreact to your puppy if it squeals after the vaccinations. Attempts to "baby" it will only make things worse. Gentle soothing and reassurance are all that is needed. If you are uncomfortable being in the room with the puppy when the vaccinations are given, ask the doctor if you may quietly leave before the vaccinations are administered.

During this socialization period, it is critical to start introducing your puppy to as many necessary interactions as possible. For example, consider giving your puppy a bath, clipping its nails, picking up and handling its feet, putting the puppy on its back until it lies still, brushing its teeth, taking food and toys away without it growling, cleaning its ears, opening its mouth, and brushing its coat. Have your doctor show you how to perform these procedures. Your puppy needs to be tolerant of these procedures without resisting or acting aggressive. It is critical to the well-being of your pet that you can perform necessary procedures without fear of attack. These procedures take only a few seconds each to perform and will help you bond with your new puppy. Performing these procedures regularly during the 8- to 12-week critical period of socialization will help make your puppy a great dog as he matures.

Common Owner Concerns

Q: I've heard many people say the ideal time to buy a puppy is before 6 weeks of age. Others say I should wait until the puppy is several months old and has had most of his vaccinations. Is there a best time for buying a new puppy?

A: There is no right age to buy a puppy, but there are several problems that can occur if a puppy is purchased at too young or too old an age.

If the puppy is too young when purchased (under 6 weeks of age), it may not have learned what it means to be a puppy and may have trouble interacting with other dogs as it ages. If purchased too old (12 weeks or later), the puppy may not have been socialized to interact properly with humans.

Some breeders feel that once a puppy is weaned (i.e., no longer nursing the mother) he should be placed in a home. Weaning, while important, is not the deciding factor. (Some unethical breeders wean puppies at 3-4 weeks of age to allow the mother dog to produce more litters.) Wait until at least 6-8 weeks of age; your puppy should be weaned by then and will be a better adjusted pet as well.

The environment the puppy is coming from as well as the environment you will provide are more important than an arbitrary age. Puppies that have been properly socialized by others will behave properly in your new home if you continue to work on socializing them. A puppy reared in a "puppy mill" environment with no handling or discipline is likely to have difficulty socializing, especially if he is purchased at an older age. Most doctors recommend buying a puppy between 6 and 8 weeks old. This lets you, the new owner, start training the puppy properly during its critical learning stages. It also allows you to be the one to comfort him during veterinary visits and ensures proper medical attention and immunizations without needing to depend on a third party.

Chapter 7
Selecting a Groomer

. . . .

After selecting the proper puppy and the right veterinarian, selecting a groomer is the next important task for owners of the breeds of puppies which require regular grooming. These breeds include poodles, Bichon frises, some terriers, cocker spaniels, Lhasa apsos, and Shih Tzus. These dogs require regular grooming every 4-8 weeks. Owners can consult various textbooks which are available to learn proper grooming techniques and purchase the proper grooming equipment themselves, but most choose to take their pets to a professional for their regular "haircut."

If your veterinarian offers grooming services, this is the ideal place to take your puppy. You have already established a good relationship there and have developed a rapport and degree of trust with the doctor and the staff. Additionally, the doctor is available in the event that sedatives might be needed to make it easier to groom your pet (which shouldn't be necessary if you've done a good job of socializing your puppy and have taken it to obedience classes). Also, if the groomer detects any medical problems, these can be treated that same day by your veterinarian, which saves you another trip and expense if your pet is groomed elsewhere. If you decide to have your pet groomed at the veterinary hospital, make sure you tour the grooming area and meet the groomer. As with your doctor, you need to be comfortable with the person who will be doing the grooming.

HOME GROOMING ....

Home grooming, including daily brushing or combing and regular trimming of puppy's nails, is a regular part of puppy care. While you can pay the veterinarian to trim the nails, it's not a hard procedure to learn and will increase the bonding between pet and owner. Have the doctor show you how on one of your visits.

There are several brands of nail trimmers you can purchase from your veterinarian or local pet store. Rescoe nail trimmers are suitable for small breed dogs; for larger breeds (20 pounds or more of adult body weight) I would recommend Miller's Forge trimmers. Also be sure you purchase some type of styptic in case the nails are trimmed too short and bleed. Powders, sticks, or liquids are available.

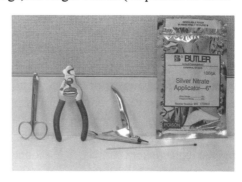

While many owners want to take their new puppies for a grooming as soon as possible, it is best to wait until at least 4 months of age. That way, your puppy will have had all of its puppy vaccinations and be fully protected against disease. Because grooming is slightly stressful, and because many pets are housed in close quarters at many grooming shops, the chance for disease spread can be high. Waiting until your puppy is vaccinated can go a long way in preventing illness.

While you're waiting until your puppy has completed its series of vaccinations, you can accustom it to what it can expect at the groomer's. Daily brushing or combing, along with an occasional (every 1-2 weeks) bath, and a nail trim every 1-2 months, will get the puppy used to these procedures.

Selecting a groomer involves the same steps as selecting a veterinarian. Asking friends or family members for a reference is quick and easy. If your veterinarian doesn't offer grooming,

When you trim the nails, avoid the quick, which is the pink area of the nail representing the artery, vein, and nerve of the nail.

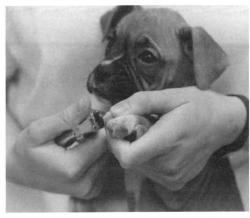

The quick is easily seen in white nails but difficult to see in dark nails. As a rule, I like to leave the nails a little long so that the animal isn't "quicked" and doesn't bleed.

Brushing or combing should be done on a daily basis to remove dead hair and prevent matting

All puppies should be trained to accept nail trimming.

of the coat. I usually use a comb for fine-haired puppies (poodles, Bichon frises) and a brush for thicker-haired puppies (retrievers, collies). Check with your doctor or groomer for further tips on daily grooming for your pets.

he or she or the staff can be an excellent source for a referral (they may even be able to tell you who to avoid). Using the yellow pages to locate a groomer is also convenient, but may not lead you to the best groomer. Finally, locating nearby salons as you drive in your neighborhood will give you several possible choices as well.

After collecting names of possible groomers from these sources, it's time to do some investigating. Visit several of the grooming salons. Make sure you meet the actual person who will be doing the grooming. If you pick up any bad vibes from the groomer, this is not the place to have your puppy groomed. If your first impression of the facility is unfavorable—for example, if it is dirty or smelly—leave.

Inquire about vaccination protocols. Does the shop require all animals to be vaccinated? Do they verify this by asking you to bring in the vaccination records in writing or by calling your doctor to confirm the vaccinations? A grooming salon that doesn't require vaccinations should not receive as high a ranking as one that does. Many do not, and it may be hard to find one that is this stringent; once again, veterinarians who offer grooming services maintain higher standards than grooming shops. Fees are important, but less so than the feel you get for the shop and the groomer.

When leaving your puppy for grooming, make sure you and the groomer communicate clearly about what type of cut you want for your puppy. If you don't know anything about the various grooming options, ask about different clips before you ever pick a groomer. Make sure the groomer clearly explains

your options and shows a willingness to work with you as a first-time client.

When you pick your puppy up after its first grooming, don't panic if it looks a bit different than you expected. As with any new hair style, you never know exactly what the finished product will look like until you see it. If the puppy doesn't look quite the way you thought it would, realize that it may take a few tries for any groomer to understand your desires. Communication before and after the grooming is important so that the groomer can rectify the situation as needed.

Many groomers like to put powder in a dog's ears after

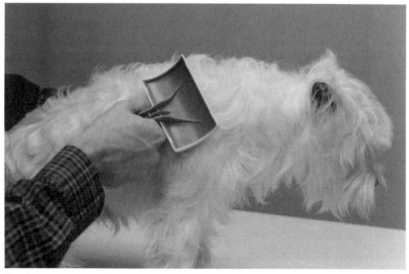

Brushing your puppy should be a part of his daily routine.

bathing in an attempt to absorb excess moisture. Most veterinary dermatologists agree that powder is not needed and may increase the chance of ear infections. Ear cleaning solutions are available from your veterinarian that properly dry a pet's ear without causing ear infections. Be sure to discuss this with your veterinarian and groomer.

Finally, you may want to avoid the additional expense of a flea dip (unless the groomer sees fleas and requires it). First, many groomers use the cheapest shampoo and dip available; you may be paying for something that is ineffective. Second, if your puppy is taking ProSpot as prescribed by your doctor for flea control, it would be harmful and possibly fatal to dip the puppy.

Make sure your groomer is aware of any medical conditions your dog has to make the experience a safe one. Also, if your veterinarian recommends a certain grooming shampoo, be sure to bring that along for the groomer to use. Any groomer who refuses these requests is one to take off your list.

Common Owner Concerns

Q: Is it really necessary to pay a groomer to cut my puppy's hair? It seems like I could do it a lot cheaper.

A: It is not essential that you hire someone to clip your pet's coat. However, most owners have no formal training in grooming and don't have the time to learn or the money for the equipment, although the equipment is not expensive. If you wish to learn to groom your pet yourself, check to see if a local community college offers courses on the subject. Your pet store probably has books on grooming that can teach you the proper cut for your breed of dog. Make sure that your puppy is groomed at least every 1-2 months; if you don't mind the investment of time and money, you can learn to give a basic cut yourself.

Q: Our groomer mentioned that our dog needs to be sedated the next time she comes in for grooming due to her aggressiveness. I'm concerned about tranquilizing her; is this really necessary?

A: Sedating the animal can make it easier for the groomer to do his job. It is rarely necessary, however. If a sedative needs to be given, make sure you discuss this with your dog's doctor first. Don't let the groomer administer any medication to your pet without your doctor's OK. Teaching puppies at an early age to allow nail trimming and brushing will do a lot to prevent the need for tranquilizers at her grooming visit.

Q: The last time our dog was groomed he got a clipper burn. The groomer said it wasn't his fault, but I think he got overly aggressive with the clippers. Do I need to look for another groomer?

A: "Clipper burn" is a term used when a dog develops an area of acute moist dermatitis (a "hot spot") after grooming. The cause can be from the clippers, but more than likely there is another reason. Possibly your dog struggled during the grooming and was shaved too closely in one area.

If your dog has not been groomed in a while, the short hair produced by the recent grooming probably itched, he scratched it, it itched more, he scratched more, and he caused the abrasion or "hot spot." I wouldn't suggest switching groomers if you have not had any other problems. Make sure your dog is groomed on a regular basis as recommended by the groomer or your veterinarian. If future clipper burns occur despite regular grooming, it may be the fault of the groomer.

Chapter 8

Spaying or Breeding

$\mathbf{A}$ decision every pet owner must face is whether or not to breed his pet. This is an important decision and it should only be made by an informed pet owner.

Breeding

There is no question that some pet owners would like to breed their dogs when they get older. An important thing to consider, however, is the motivation behind the desire to breed. Three questions must be asked by every owner prior to breeding his pet:

1. Why do I want to breed my dog?

2. Is my dog of breeding quality?

3. Can I afford to breed my dog?

Why Do I Want To Breed My Dog?

If you desire to breed your puppy when it gets older, is your motivation financial? Do you expect to make money on the puppies that result from the breeding? If money is your motivation, you should be aware that most owners who breed their dogs rarely make any significant amount of money. Some owners, in fact, lose a considerable amount of money due to the cost of veterinary care for the mother and puppies and feeding the litter. Also, if you own the female dog and she has only one puppy, you are almost guaranteed not to make any money.

Do you want to breed your dog so your children can learn about the "birds and the bees"?

Dogs rarely give birth at a convenient time; most children aren't awake at two in the morning. How will your children act when they see the blood and fluids normally passed during the birthing process? What if the mother has problems during the delivery of the puppies? Will your children be able to understand and handle the pain and trauma involved with a complicated birth? Some dogs, especially first-time mothers of smaller breeds, are nervous and easily stressed while giving birth if they have an audience. Dogs can prolong labor until you and the kids go back to bed. Additionally, some dogs that are stressed will actually kill and eat their newborn puppies. This can be traumatic for children and adults alike. Most children can learn about the birthing experience through better means than watching their dog deliver puppies.

Should My Dog Be Bred?

Most pets are not the ideal standards of the breed. Was your pet sold as a "pet quality" or "breeding quality" puppy? Some pets have medical or behavioral problems that might be passed to the offspring. Most breeders will not allow their dogs to breed with a family pet, even if it is purebred, unless it is a champion and has won many contests. Does your dog have an outstanding pedigree? Is he or she registered? If you feel that your dog is a

---

BEFORE YOU BREED YOUR PET . . . .

If after careful consideration, you have decided to breed your puppy when he or she reaches breeding age (2-5 years of age is preferred by many veterinarians), consider the following points before firmly committing to this project:

• •➡ Is your pet healthy? Only healthy dogs that are free from genetic disorders should be bred. A veterinary visit prior to breeding is essential. Of course, your pet should be current on all vaccinations, be dewormed as needed, be free of internal and external parasites, and take a heartworm preventative medication.

• •➡ Does your pet have any hereditary defects? Any pet with a condition which is known or suspected to be hereditary in nature

perfect specimen, consult with your veterinarian to make sure it does not have any genetic defects. This can be expensive, but it is necessary. A visit with a local breeder will confirm if your puppy is an outstanding representative of the breed.

Can I Afford to Breed My Dog?

Assuming there are no medical problems with the mother, the birthing process, or the puppies, the minimum cost for providing veterinary care for a female dog and an average litter of five puppies that will be sold at 8 weeks of age is approximately $250. This does not include breeding, boarding, and testing costs. If the mother needs a Caesarean section in order to deliver the puppies, add another $500-$1,000 to that cost. For each sick puppy, add another $300 or so. Since most owners will get no more than $150-$250 per puppy, you can see that breeding dogs is usually not a money-making business. Unless you can commit to providing all the care an expectant mother and new puppies will require, seriously reconsider the idea of breeding your pet. Will you be able to provide care for a litter of puppies if you have trouble finding homes? Can you find good owners for your puppies? Even though you may think your puppies are cute and adorable, it doesn't mean you'll have buyers knocking down your door to take them.

---

should not be bred. These include but are not limited to hip, elbow, or shoulder dysplasia; demodectic mange; atopic or allergic dermatitis; monorchism; hernias; eye defects; and heart conditions.

•• ➡ Is the owner of the intended mate responsible? Even though you may not own both the male and female, you still have a responsibility to make sure the mate for your dog is healthy and free of hereditary defects.

•• ➡ What are the dog's temperament and behavior? Only well-mannered and even-tempered pets should be used for breeding.

•• ➡ Can you keep the litter of puppies if for some reason you are unable to sell them? If you answer "no," then you should not breed your dog.

Reasons Not to Breed Your Dog

In addition to all of the above arguments against breeding your male or female dog, there are medical and behavioral reasons for spaying or neutering. Malignant breast cancer occurs in about one in four unspayed female dogs, compared to a one-in-nine chance in women. The older the dog is when she is spayed, the greater the chance of breast cancer. Puppies spayed before their first heat, which occurs at approximately 6 months of age, have almost no chance of developing breast cancer. After 2 years of age, dogs should still be spayed if this has not already been done, but there is no protective effect against developing breast cancer. Nevertheless, all dogs should eventually be spayed, even those that have puppies, to prevent the development of a common condition called pyometra, which is an infection (often life-threatening) of the uterus. This condition commonly develops in dogs that have never been spayed; while it usually occurs in older dogs past 8 years of age, it can occur at any time in any unspayed female dog.

During the spaying operation, the ovaries and the uterus are removed. Dogs that have been spayed will never come into heat and display the behaviors associated with the fluctuating hormone levels of intact female dogs.

Neutering of male dogs includes removal of the testicles and the vas deferens (spermatic cord). This prevents the hormonal effects seen in intact male dogs. Early neutering can prevent prostate disease and certain anal tumors as well as testicular cancer.

While most female dogs are spayed, many male dogs are not neutered. This is often due to a "castration complex" among male owners. Often the wife wants the dog neutered but the husband does not. It seems that, consciously or subconsciously, the husband identifies with the dog and equates the neutering with his own castration, which somehow lowers his masculinity. Careful discussion between both husband and wife and veterinarian can usually make the neutering process less traumatic for male pet owners.

Many owners incorrectly assume that spays and neuters are routine procedures. This is a very dangerous assumption that leads to complacency among owners and sometimes even veterinarians. Spaying and neutering are major surgical procedures. Anytime a pet is anesthetized, there is a risk of injury or even death.

The following description will help you understand what actually occurs during a spaying (ovariohysterectomy) or neutering (orchidectomy) procedure. Since your veterinarian may do things slightly differently, make sure you talk with him about the specifics of the procedure that he performs. This is definitely one time when you need to be comfortable with your choice in doctors. Do not send your pet to the lowest bidder for surgery!

1. Prior to the anesthetic, the dog is given a complete physical examination and blood tests to make sure it is healthy. Any abnormalities noted on the examination or blood tests may warrant further investigation of the problem and delay the spaying or neutering. Problems very rarely are found, but anything that might contribute to the injury or death of your pet needs to be checked out *before* an elective surgical procedure.

2. Assuming the examination and blood tests are normal, the pet will be given a sedative and usually a drug that can prevent unnecessary slowing of the heart once anesthetized. The sedative helps calm the pet and make induction of anesthesia easier. Sedatives also reduce the amount of anesthetic needed; this is wise, as the major risk involved in surgery is with the anesthesia. Sedatives also help the pet wake up smoothly from the anesthetic and may offer some postoperative pain relief.

3. The animal can be given any of several types of anesthetic. The most expensive, but also the safest, is a gas called isoflurane. Many doctors prefer this anesthetic, as the pet's depth of anesthesia can be easily regulated. Pets that become "light" (start to wake up) can be given more gas; pets that breathe a little too slowly (become too deeply anesthetized) can be given less anesthesia. Animals are usually induced with a short-acting injectable anesthetic that allows the doctor to place a tube into its trachea (windpipe) to administer the anesthetic gas. In an attempt to cut costs, lower-priced spay and neuter clinics usually will not use isoflurane gas but opt instead for the much less expensive injectable anesthetics. These injectable

anesthetics, while often safe, are not as safe as isoflurane, and the depth of anesthesia is not easily controlled. Additionally, they often wear off before the procedure ends, causing the animal to feel pain from the surgery. Finally, pets given only injectable anesthetics often wake up violently and appear drugged or "spaced out" for several hours or days after the surgery.

4. The anesthesia and surgery are monitored by a veterinary assistant and any of several machines. The machine could be a respiratory monitor, which indicates when the animal breathes, a heart monitor, which indicates heart rate, or a new device called a pulse oximeter which indicates oxygen saturation of the pet's tissues. Any of these devices, accompanied by the watchful eye of the assistant, ensure proper anesthetic depth and can alert the doctor if any problems develop during the surgical procedure.

5. During a spay procedure, the ovaries and uterus are located, clamped, and tied with absorbable suture material that will dissolve within one to two

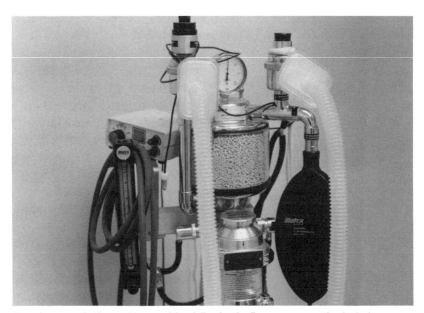

A modern anesthetic machine used for delivering isoflurane gas anesthesia during surgery. Notice the respiratory monitor (small box on the left side of the machine) which alerts the doctor of breathing pattern changes during the surgery.

months. The abdomen is sutured, usually with absorbable suture; the skin is sutured with buried (hidden) absorbable suture or visible nonabsorbable suture or stainless steel that must be removed by the doctor within seven to ten days following the surgery.

During a neuter, the testes and spermatic cord (vas deferens) are located, clamped, and tied with absorbable suture material. The skin is sutured with buried (hidden) absorbable suture or visible nonabsorbable suture or stainless steel that must

be removed by the doctor within seven to ten days following the surgery.

6. After the procedure is completed, the gas anesthetic is turned off and the animal recovers in a quiet compartment or run. The animal is usually kept overnight to ensure a quiet recovery.

As you can see, these surgeries, while common procedures, are *not* routine, and problems, though extremely rare, can arise. Make sure you are comfortable with the doctor you select to

STERILIZATION AND PET BEHAVIOR . . . .

Many owners are concerned about the behavioral changes seen in their pets after sterilization. Most of the time there will be no changes, as far as a calming effect. Remember, these surgeries occur when the pet is still a young puppy. Surgical sterilization does not change that fact, and these puppies will still be energetic and puppy-like for a long time. About 50 percent of the time, dogs that are exhibiting undesirable behaviors may have those problems corrected by neutering or spaying. These behaviors can include aggression, urine marking, and the desire to roam or fight with other dogs. Male dogs that are not sterilized can be a challenge to control unless used regularly for mating.

Spaying or neutering is best done immediately after the last set of vaccinations, at approximately 4 months of age. To prevent problems associated with the hormonal influences seen at puberty, it is best to have these surgeries done by 6 months of age. However, it is never too late to have a dog spayed or neutered, and the procedure can also be done on older pets.

perform either of these operations on your puppy. Don't be afraid to inquire as to the exact specifics of the procedure, type of anesthesia used, type of monitoring done during the surgery, and any other questions you may have.

Aftercare of the pet is extremely important. Your doctor should review discharge instructions with you. The pet must be kept quiet; this means physical activity must be kept to a minimum (short leash walks, no running, jumping, or hard play) to prevent dehiscence. Dehiscence occurs when excess pressure or tension is put on the suture line; if this occurs, the wound dehisces or breaks open and must be resutured. This is a serious complication; wounds that break open are susceptible to infection. Additionally, abdominal contents, such as fat (usually) or intestines (rarely) can hang out of the open incision and can result in infection, shock, or even death if not treated immediately. If you have trouble keeping your pet quiet at home, consult with the doctor for advice. Some puppies, being active and playful, may need to be sedated until the sutures are removed. Others should be boarded for a week or confined to a cage at home during this recovery time.

Common Owner Concerns

Q: I've been told that all female dogs need to go through at least one heat or even be bred prior to being spayed. Shouldn't I wait until my dog has a litter of puppies before spaying her?

A: At one time, the general consensus was that all female dogs should go through at least one heat period prior to spaying. Some doctors even recommended letting a dog have at least one litter before spaying. Now we know the many benefits of early spaying, including the significant reduction in breast cancer in dogs that are spayed before their first heat. While some people still believe the old school of thought, realize that there are no benefits to putting off spaying your dog. Unless your dog is a registered champion and you have the patience and finances to handle the breeding and raising of puppies, get your puppy spayed between 4 and 6 months of age.

Q: Our puppy has had a bout of what her doctor calls puppy vaginitis. He recommended letting her go through one heat cycle to help cure this problem. Does that make sense?

A: Puppy vaginitis is a rare condition in puppies. It is felt that many puppies will self-cure after their first heat due to hormonal changes in the reproductive tract. Medication controls the problem until that time. While we desire all puppies to be spayed before their first heat, occasionally an exception is made. The chance of breast cancer in puppies that have one heat is slightly increased; if your doctor feels it is in your puppy's best interest to have one heat due to the

---

OVARIAN REMNANT SYNDROME ....

Occasionally a spayed dog will still go through a heat cycle. Assuming the operation was performed correctly, the most common cause of this problem is ovarian remnant syndrome.

During the spaying procedure, the ovaries are clamped, cut, and removed, and the stump where the ovaries were attached is tied with suture material. While this is usually a straightforward procedure, in rare cases there might be microscopic amounts of ovarian tissue left in the stump. If this is the case, after spaying, that microscopic tissue will enlarge and function as another ovary. This seems more common in large breed dogs that are spayed later in life; these dogs often have a large amount of fat in their ovarian areas, and it is difficult to remove all of the tissue in this case. This is another reason to have dogs spayed between 4 and 6 months of age.

The solution is simply to do an exploratory surgery and remove any remaining ovarian tissue; the doctor may want to send this tissue off for a biopsy to confirm that it is ovarian tissue and make sure no cancer is involved. While this does result in an extra cost for the owner, the extra ovarian tissue must be removed to prevent future heat cycles and possible health problems.

vaginitis, follow his advice and have her spayed right after her heat cycle.

Q: Is the heat cycle in dogs the same as the menstrual cycle in women? My dog's heat seems to last longer than the typical period in women.

A: The heat cycle in dogs is very different from the menstrual cycle in women. Most dogs have approximately two heat cycles each year, versus approximately one menstrual cycle each month in women. This means that the reproductive tract is "quiet" or less active in dogs than people.

With women, bleeding occurs as the menstrual cycle is ending, after the uterus, primed under hormonal influence for possible pregnancy, sheds its blood-rich lining. In dogs, bleeding is seen before the uterus is prepared for pregnancy; this indi-cates the start of the heat cycle. A dog usually is in heat for three weeks: the first week there is the bleeding, the second week the female will usually stand to be bred, and the third week the dog is going out of heat. As with women, these are textbook num-bers for the average dog; your pet may differ without being abnormal. Many puppies have a silent heat that is not recognized by the owners. Some dogs, particularly the smaller, cleaner breeds, may fastidiously groom themselves to where the owner never notices vaginal bleeding.

Dogs can get pregnant at any time during the typical three weeks of heat. If you plan on breeding your dog and you notice more than two heats each year, or you never notice a heat cycle, these could indicate prob-lems that need to be checked by the doctor.

Chapter 9

Common Puppy Behavior Problems

· ·

Without question, the two most common behavioral problems new puppy owners face are housebreaking and destructive chewing. Just about every new puppy owner has to deal with these problems sooner or later, so take comfort in knowing that you are not alone.

The difficult thing for owners to understand is that most behavior problems are not necessarily abnormal behaviors. An example of an abnormal behavior would be a dog acting self-destructively, such as constantly chewing at a spot on its leg until the spot becomes raw. Most of the behavior problems owners notice in their puppies are normal behaviors for the puppy, just not appreciated or allowed by owners. Like it or not, a puppy that is eliminating throughout the house or chewing furniture is engaging in normal, although unacceptable, behavior.

In trying to prevent abnormal elimination and chewing, realize that most puppies learn quickly if you will just be patient with them. Puppies have short attention spans; learning is difficult, requires a lot of energy, and repetition is important. When possible, praise goes a lot further than punishment.

Housetraining

Probably the biggest concern owners have with a new puppy is housetraining. As with potty training a child, it is important that puppies be housetrained right from the start. The older the pet becomes, the harder it will be to housetrain.

With most dogs, housetraining is a simple task. Most puppies learn housetraining readily if the owners perform the task properly. Some other puppies are a bit slower; as with toilet training children, each puppy will learn at its own pace, a pace that can't be rushed by impatient owners.

The following is a basic discussion of housetraining; your puppy may deviate from it and need additional help. Work with your veterinarian to establish proper training methods early.

There are several rules to follow when attempting to housetrain a puppy, and adhering to these rules will go a long way in decreasing the time it takes to properly housetrain your new friend.

Rule 1. It is better to praise than punish. Puppies, like people, learn more with praise than with punishment. This is not to suggest that puppies should never be punished, only that if owners have a choice, praise is always preferred.

Rule 2. In order for punishment to work, it must be initiated promptly, it must "fit the crime," and it should be of sufficient duration to correct the behavior. Punishment that lasts for too short a period is ineffective; punishment that lasts too long is cruel and also ineffective.

Prompt punishment means that the puppy must be caught "in the act" or within 30 seconds of the act. This is impossible for most owners. Often the puppy has an accident out of the owner's sight; punishment of the inappropriate elimination then is ineffective. Taking a puppy over to the spot, scolding, hitting, and rubbing the nose of the puppy in the area will not correct the problem but in fact will encourage the behavior and make the problem worse.

Puppies need to eliminate:
- after eating
- after playing
- after waking (from a nap or the previous night's sleep)
- before going to sleep at night

Taking advantage of these times when we know the puppy needs to eliminate will greatly improve the chance of success with housetraining.

When you take the puppy outside, it is critical to the success of the housetraining program that you stay with the puppy. Remember, you want to catch the puppy doing something right so you can lavish extensive praise on it. Leaving a puppy outside on its own reduces your chance of rewarding it for proper behavior.

Staying with the puppy may mean waiting 10-20 minutes before it eliminates; this is not easy and obviously takes time. However, it is necessary in order to give the puppy time to find a suitable spot for its elimination. After 10-20 minutes, if the puppy hasn't eliminated, it probably doesn't need to and can be brought back inside.

When the puppy eliminates for you, lavish a lot of praise on it. A small food treat (a morsel of its food or low-fat puppy biscuit) can help reinforce this good behavior. The puppy learns that when it eliminates outside, it gets rewarded. When it eliminates inside, there is no reward or food and sometimes a punishment as well.

One caution about food treats: we don't want to create obesity. A typical puppy biscuit can easily be broken into 5-10 small rewards. The common puppy biscuits often have 100 calories or more per biscuit; talk with your veterinarian about purchasing low-fat treats your puppy will enjoy. The point in using food treats for any kind of training is to reward proper behavior, not to fill the puppy's tummy!

When the puppy eliminates inside, he should be gently punished only if caught in the act. A firm but loud "no" or "stop" is all the punishment that is usually needed to be effective.

When you are away from the house, or when you cannot watch the puppy closely (i.e., you're asleep, cooking, getting dressed for work), the puppy should be confined, ideally to a small kennel or crate. Work with your veterinarian in choosing a crate of the appropriate size. Food and water can be left in the crate, but once again heed your doctor's advice.

As the puppy improves its housetraining habits, you will gradually start to give it the run of the house (unless you make it an outdoor dog). As you give it access to the house, room by room, keep an eye on it every so often. Accidents will happen occasionally, but if the puppy begins a regular pattern of elimination in other rooms it may need a refresher course in housetraining.

Adherence to a fairly strict schedule works best. Owners whose schedule varies from day to day often have a harder time housebreaking their new puppies. Interestingly, adhering to a fairly routine schedule can help prevent many behavior problems commonly seen in dogs.

Most puppies will be fully housetrained by their last puppy visit, which occurs at about 4 months of age. Some puppies learn faster and will be housetrained sooner. Occasionally, a rare individual will take longer to housetrain or never learn proper eliminative behavior. These "slower" pets seem to be the smaller breeds (under 10 pounds of adult weight) which are often bred to retain "juvenile" characteristics.

Destructive Chewing

It is normal behavior for puppies to chew on various objects, including their owners' fingers and toes! Puppies, like young children, investigate their environment through their mouths. Additionally, puppies are "teething" until they have all of their permanent or adult teeth, at about 6 months of age. Finally,

some breeds of dogs are "mouth oriented," such as retrievers, and need to chew a lot. Puppies and dogs which are overly energetic and don't get a chance for regular exercise may use their teeth to release this extra energy (running in the backyard by itself is not adequate exercise for any pet). Puppies that experience environmental stress or "frustration" may also become destructive chewers.

A common concern of owners is how to get the puppy to stop chewing on them, their clothing, and their furniture. Although chewing is a normal behavior that cannot be stopped, we can direct the puppy's chewing toward acceptable objects.

First, family members should discourage the puppy's chewing. Some may find it cute that the puppy chews on them, but this "cute" behavior can easily develop into aggressive biting as the puppy matures.

Second, careful selection of chewing toys is needed. Owners should not offer puppies old shoes or socks; your puppy can't tell the difference between an old shoe and your new, expensive pair.

Avoid tug-of-war games that encourage aggressiveness, biting, and chewing.

TOYS ....

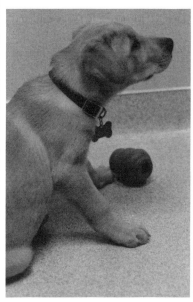

Puppies love toys, and it seems most owners love buying toys for their puppies. Offer a variety of playthings to your pet, and keep the following points in mind:

••➡ Make sure the size of the item fits the size of the dog; don't offer a puppy anything that can be easily swallowed or an item that might be big but can easily be chewed into smaller pieces that can be swallowed.

••➡ Avoid stuffed toys that are easily destroyed and leave only the stuffing behind. Many puppies can develop intestinal obstructions from the stuffing. Also avoid toys with pieces that can easily come off (such as eyes on a doll) and be swallowed.

••➡ Puppies are teething for the first six months of their lives and *need* to chew; it's better they chew on toys than on you or the furniture!

••➡ In addition to toys, small amounts of rawhide are acceptable, as are pig ears that are available in pet stores.

••➡ Stay away from things that are harmful, such as pig or cow hooves that can easily break puppy and dog teeth.

••➡ If you want to offer real bones, ask the butcher for beef knuckle or ox tail bones. Many butchers also can supply beef femurs (leg bones). Chicken, steak, and pork bones are easily splintered and can cause problems.

There are many acceptable chew toys. Rawhide, offered in small amounts, is acceptable and considered safe for dogs.

The Nylabone brand of toys offers a variety of shapes and sizes that also help control periodontal disease, similar to daily rawhide treats.

Kong brand toys are also ideal for correcting chewing misbehavior. Kong toys are hollow, strong rubber toys with an opening at one end. The toy can be smeared with a small amount of peanut butter and stuffed with several food treats. Some of the treats should be a small size that will easily fall out as the puppy plays with the toy. Other treats should be oversized and stuffed in the Kong toy. These treats will not easily come out and the puppy will spend a large amount of time biting and chewing at the toy (and not at the owner or furniture) in an attempt to remove the oversized treats. Some behavior specialists recommend purchasing a half dozen or so Kongs, loading them with treats, and hiding them in various places in the house so that the puppy spends a lot of time seeking out the treats and working to remove them from the toys, behavior similar to that of dogs in the wild.

When your puppy bites you, discipline the puppy with a firm "no" and then give it an appropriate chew toy to satisfy its desire to chew.

Juvenile Fear Period

Some puppies, from about 6-18 months of age, will go through a "fear" period that may last a few months. These puppies seem to be afraid of objects they are accustomed to, such as the garbage can, lawn mower, and even the owner! With time, most of these puppies will resolve their fear of these objects. Reinforcing proper behavior with another training (obedience) class at this time is helpful.

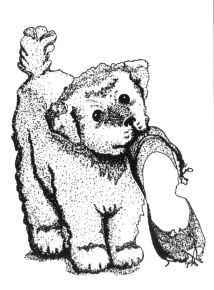

Common Owner Concerns

• •

Q: Our little cocker spaniel puppy urinates whenever she gets excited. Even though we yell at her to stop, she continues the behavior. Will this ever end?

A: Your puppy does not seem to be experiencing a housebreaking problem but rather another type of eliminative problem, actually two problems. The first is typical of puppies in general and cocker spaniels in particular, that of urinating when excited. Puppies will often "grow out of this" as they enter puberty. Try to avoid exciting her.

Your puppy may also be exhibiting submissive urination. By punishing her when she urinates as she gets excited, you're only making the problem worse. Punishment does not work with excited or submissive urinary problems. Avoid punishment when she urinates. If she urinates when excited, ignore her and do something else. By ignoring her, you're removing the stimulus to make her urinate. Avoiding punishment for a few weeks may help the submissive urinary problem. See your veterinarian for other suggestions before the problem gets out of hand.

Q: Our puppy is an 8-month-old male. We were thinking about breeding him, but he is urinating all over the house. He is housebroken, but he likes to lift his leg on our good chairs. Should we have him neutered?

A: Neutering is 50 to 60 percent effective in eliminating house soiling (urine marking) in intact male dogs. Assuming that the elimination is marking behavior related to hormone levels, neutering would most likely solve the problem. Neutering should also be done to reduce the risk of prostatic disease and the elimination of the chance for testicular cancer. It's never too late to have your dog neutered, regardless of its age!

Chapter 10

Common Puppyhood Diseases

· ·

While preventing illness is every owner's goal, your puppy may require veterinary attention for an illness at some point in its life. Most puppyhood illnesses are mild and not life-threatening, as is true of many childhood diseases. Early diagnosis and treatment are important in help-ing your puppy make a quick and smooth recovery. Illness is hard on puppies; the sooner they recover from an illness, the happier you will both feel.

This section talks about some of the most common conditions affecting puppies.

Viral Diseases
· ·

Distemper

Distemper is a highly contagious viral disease of dogs, mainly affecting unvaccinated puppies. The disease was reported in Europe as early as the mid 1700s.

Distemper is related to the human measles virus. While dogs will not get measles nor people contract distemper, this similarity in viruses is useful in allowing very young puppies to be vaccinated against distemper using a human measles vaccine.

Distemper virus is shed in the feces, saliva, urine, and discharge from the eyes and nostrils of infected dogs. Aerosol and droplet exposure are the most common routes of infection.

Unvaccinated or partially vaccinated dogs that are exposed to distemper virus may show signs within two weeks of exposure. These signs include fever, weight loss, anorexia, diarrhea, difficulty breathing, tremors, and seizures. The animal usually dies within one to three weeks after developing these signs. Fever, coughing, and nasal and eye discharge are the most common symptoms. Secondary infections, which occur commonly, cause pneumonia and a pustular (pimple-looking) dermatitis on the abdomen (which most owners mistakenly assume is the result of ant bites).

Involvement of the nervous system is common in many dogs with distemper and is often what prevents recovery from the infection. Young puppies are especially prone to developing nervous system signs, including behavioral changes, seizures, paralysis, muscle twitching, and "chewing gum" fits.

Diagnosis is usually made by the veterinarian based on the history and clinical signs. Most puppies with signs of distemper have had no vaccinations; others have had only a part of the vacci-

nation series completed. Certain diagnostic tests aid in the diagnosis of distemper. The best one is analysis of the cerebral spinal fluid, which bathes the brain and spinal cord. Unfortunately, most owners will not pay $100 or more for this test. Blood tests can be used to check for antibodies to the distemper virus but are not 100 percent accurate and can be misleading. While a positive diagnostic test can be helpful, blood tests usually are not needed since so few diseases cause signs that would be confused with canine distemper in young, unvaccinated puppies.

As one veterinary publication has stated, the lack of effective antiviral treatment creates the need for supportive care and a guarded-to-poor prognosis. All that veterinarians can do is keep the puppy well hydrated, fed, and warm, and treat or ideally prevent any secondary infections such as pneumonia, which is very common. Intravenous antibiotics and fluids, force-feeding, and a warm environment are used during the course of therapy if treatment is elected. If there are neurological signs, such as seizures, the prognosis is very grim. Most owners will euthanize puppies once neurological signs develop. While some puppies can be saved, most owners will not spend the money (often $500-$1,000) on hospitalization for a puppy with a poor chance of recovery and the possibility of lifelong complications such as epilepsy. Vaccination is very effective in preventing the disease. Most vaccinated dogs that are exposed to distemper virus develop a short-lived infection without showing signs of illness. Puppies 6 weeks of age are vaccinated with a measles vaccine. The puppy often has maternal antibodies he received from his mother that would interfere with his ability to form antibodies to a canine distemper vaccine. He is able to develop protective antibodies to the measles vaccine; however the protection is transient and a distemper vaccine should be given in two to three weeks (usually at 8 weeks of age, the time when he starts his puppy vaccinations).

Parvo Virus

Parvo virus is another devastating and potentially fatal disease most commonly afflicting young puppies. Discovered in the 1970s, this is a relatively new disease in dogs. It is similar to a viral disease of cats, feline pan-leukopenia virus. In fact, until a vaccine specific for parvo virus was produced, dogs were vaccinated against parvo virus with the cat panleukopenia vaccine.

Unvaccinated or partially vaccinated puppies are very susceptible to infection with parvo virus. The virus is contracted by contact with infected feces; people, toys, food bowls, and insects may also spread the virus if they transport infected feces to the puppy.

Clinical signs are seen within seven to fourteen days after infection. Vomiting, often severe, is seen first, followed by diarrhea which is often very bloody. Lack of appetite, severe depression, and dehydration occur rapidly, often within 24 hours after vomiting. Temperatures are often elevated. Some young puppies may develop a cardiac form of the disease, in which case the only sign is sudden death from heart failure. This condition is not as commonly seen as when parvo virus was first discovered, since most puppies are vaccinated.

The doctor can make a presumptive diagnosis based on history and clinical signs in a susceptible puppy. Additionally, an in-office test for parvo virus is now available. Blood tests and fecal analysis for the virus are also available at outside laboratories.

Treatment is aggressive and supportive. Death is often due to dehydration or secondary bacterial infection and septicemia; therefore large amounts of fluids and antibiotics are given intravenously. Despite what many owners have heard, when treated early and aggressively most

---

WHEN TO CALL THE DOCTOR. . . . .

As a new puppy owner, you probably worry at the slightest thing that seems wrong. Don't feel bad: you're not alone. The following information may help you know when to call the doctor.

What's normal:
- An occasional sneeze
- An occasional cough
- One episode of vomiting or diarrhea, if no blood is seen and the puppy acts normal
- Mild shaking when asleep
- One skipped meal if the puppy seems normal otherwise
- A small amount of clear discharge from the eyes if the eyes are not red
- An occasional itch

What's not
(Call your veterinarian **immediately**!):
- A puppy that's sluggish, slow to wake up, or lethargic
- A puppy that shows no interest in several types of food —canned, dry, human baby food
- Red eyes, closed eyes, any eye discharge that is not clear
- Excessive scratching
- Shaking the head excessively
- More than one bout of vomiting or diarrhea
- Blood in the vomit or stool
- Abnormal size or shape to the abdomen
- Rapid breathing or difficulty breathing
- Tumors, lumps, or bumps seen or felt on the puppy
- Blood coming from any body opening

puppies with parvo virus can be saved. What was once a devastating and almost always fatal disease can now be treated successfully. Unfortunately, the average cost for treatment can easily run $500 or more, and not every owner can commit to this amount of money. With early and aggressive treatment, most puppies will live. Attempting to cut corners and save a few dollars on anything less than all-out aggressive therapy is likely to be unsuccessful and a waste of money. All puppies should be vaccinated for this disease as part of their puppy vaccination program.

Corona Virus

Corona virus is another gastrointestinal virus that was discovered in the early 1970s. Like parvo virus, it is also highly contagious and spread by contact with feces from an infected dog. Clinical signs are seen within one to four days of exposure.

Symptoms are similar to that of parvo virus, although not usually as severe. Vomiting may be seen. Diarrhea occurs suddenly and is most often orange in color (unlike the bloody red color of parvo virus), very fetid in odor, and rarely contains blood. The

animal may also experience loss of appetite and lethargy; fever may or may not be present.

Treatment is similar to that for parvo virus but is not usually as involved or expensive. Older dogs may only need mild treatment. Since puppies are more prone to dehydration and infection, most of them are treated in the hospital with IV fluids and antibiotics.

A vaccine is available for corona virus. Some doctors do not routinely vaccinate against this disease because it is not prevalent in their area. You should discuss the need for vaccination against corona virus with your doctor. The vaccine is inexpensive and preferred to treatment.

Kennel Cough

Kennel cough, or more correctly infectious tracheobronchitis, is probably the most common infectious disease seen in puppies. As the name implies, the disease is an infection of the trachea and bronchi; the trachea is the "throat" and the bronchi are the major airway tubes leading from the trachea into the lungs. Kennel cough is so named because the disease is commonly seen when dogs are closely crowded together, as in pet stores, when boarding at a kennel, or at dog shows.

Kennel cough can be caused by a bacterium named bordetella (related to the bacterium that causes whooping cough in children), a virus (parainfluenza), a mycoplasma, or any combination of these. Kennel cough is similar to a cold in humans (many owners call this a "puppy cold"), although it can be much more serious. It is a highly contagious disease of puppies, and signs are seen within three to nine days after infection.

Kennel cough is fairly easily diagnosed by the characteristic cough, or "honking," it produces. You may think your puppy is choking or gagging, as the cough is a dry cough from deep in the throat. The cough is worse at night, when the puppy gets excited, or when pressure is applied to the throat, as when walking on a leash.

Kennel cough is treated with a combination of antibiotics, corticosteroids, and cough suppressants. The antibiotics will kill the bordetella bacterium but obviously will not kill the parainfluenza virus. Nevertheless, the antibiotics are used in kennel cough because we don't always know if the bacterium, virus, or

both are causing the disease. Also, we don't want the trachea and bronchi to get so irritated that secondary bacteria set up shop and cause pneumonia. The corticosteroids relieve the inflammation in the throat and help lessen the cough. Cough suppressants are used in cases where the coughing is severe; they often make the puppy slightly drowsy as well, which further helps suppress the cough. Because they are expensive, they are not used in all cases.

There are several ways to prevent kennel cough. Several vaccines exist, including an intranasal nose drop and an injectable vaccine. The intranasal form is preferred by many veterinarians for several reasons. First, it is slightly bothersome to the puppy but is not painful to administer; the injectable vaccine seems to cause pain in many puppies. Second, immunity develops quicker with the intranasal form. Finally, since the bacterium and virus enter through the nasal and oral passages, it makes sense to administer the vaccine there and get a lot of local immunity (as with the human polio vaccine).

Common sense also helps prevent the diseases. Try to limit your puppy's exposure to other dogs until it has been fully vaccinated (by 4 months of age). This means avoiding grooming until that age, and avoiding boarding your dog if possible. When boarding your pet or having it groomed, make sure the facility is clean, has adequate ventilation, and requires proof of veterinarian-administered vaccinations of all pets. Many facilities don't require owners to show proof of vaccination, and this is just inviting disease. Try to avoid low-cost shot clinics, especially the parking lot mobile clinics, where the vaccination status of the many pets that are crowded into a confined area is often unknown.

Most veterinary facilities that offer boarding or grooming have strict admittance requirements.

Modern veterinary hospitals also have expensive but effective ventilation systems for their kennel areas; constant air movement drastically decreases the spread of infectious disease. Pets must have been examined and vaccinated by a veterinarian before a pet can be admitted for boarding or grooming. While some clients object to this because it increases the cost, most clients are happy to know that their pet will be safe from infectious disease. While no vaccine, even the kennel cough vaccine, is always 100 percent effective, regular vaccinations and adequate ventilation are essential in minimizing the exposure of your puppy to infectious diseases.

Bacterial Diseases

. . . .

Pyoderma

Pyoderma literally means "pus in the skin." Pyoderma is a fancy term for a bacterial infection of the skin, most often a staph infection. "Puppy pyoderma" is a common disease and can take two forms.

The first is superficial pyoderma, often called juvenile impetigo. This is a mild disease

and is usually seen in large breed puppies between 1 and 3 months old. Most commonly the abdomen and groin are affected. Small, itchy red bumps called papules first appear; the papules quickly turn into pustules, which resemble pimples. The disease is easily diagnosed; treatment involves medicated shampooing and oral antibiotics.

The second form of puppy pyoderma is a more serious condition called "puppy strangles," or moist juvenile pyoderma. Strangles usually affects short-haired breeds of puppies prior to 4 months of age. This is also a bacterial infection of the skin. The disease starts with swelling of the eyelids, lips, and chin; if not treated, the infection can spread to other areas of the body.

The affected skin is red, moist, tender, and painful. These puppies often have a fever (104 or higher), are lethargic, are eating less, and may have swollen lymph nodes in the jaw area. Treatment is with corticosteroids (to reduce the inflammation and fever) and antibiotics; topical soaks with a medicated cleanser are also prescribed.

BACTERIUM, FUNGUS, OR PARASITE...........

Puppies are commonly afflicted with skin conditions, or dermatitis. The three most common conditions are pyoderma/folliculitis (caused by bacteria), ringworm (caused by a fungus), and mange (caused by a microscopic parasite called a mite). Unfortunately, all three conditions look alike; certain lab tests must be performed to arrive at a correct diagnosis.

A skin scraping is an easily performed procedure that is used to check for mange mites. There are two types of mange: sarcoptic mange, which can be easily transmitted to owners, and demodectic mange. In some cases of sarcoptic mange, mites won't be found on the skin scraping, so the pet is treated based on the signs of the disease; with demodectic mange, mites are found 99 percent of the time on the scraping, which makes diagnosis easy.

A fungal culture is used to diagnose ringworm. A few hairs and crusts are gently removed from the pet and placed on a special culture plate; if ringworm is the cause of the problem, the fungus usually grows within seven days.

These simple tests make diagnosis and treatment of common puppy skin diseases fairly easy. Rest assured that most cases of puppy dermatitis are not serious and resolve rapidly with prompt treatment.

Allergic Diseases

• •

Atopy

Atopy, also called atopic dermatitis, is usually seen in dogs 1-3 years old. Atopy is often referred to as skin allergies. It is caused by the pet inhaling or absorbing foreign proteins (allergens) through its skin. The pet develops an allergic response to these allergens and signs of allergic dermatitis are then seen. While most pets are at least 1-3 years old, atopy is now being diagnosed in younger dogs as well.

Just like people, puppies can become allergic to any number of things. Grasses, trees, house dust, pollen, and molds are most common. Many of these pets are allergic to fleas and bacteria as well. The condition is mainly seen in parts of the country where fungus and pollen counts are a problem; the only way to cure the condition is to move to a part of the country where the prevalence of allergies is low or nonexistent!

Atopic dermatitis is usually diagnosed quite easily. Most pets with atopic dermatitis are moderately to severely itchy. Typical pets with this condition are described as "face rubbers, paw biters, and armpit scratchers."

However, pets with atopic dermatitis can itch anywhere on their bodies. The key to making this diagnosis is that with rare exception, the skin of an atopic dog is usually normal (with other dermatitis conditions the skin usually has hair loss or visible skin lesions). There are no skin lesions or hair loss in most cases of atopy. The only noticeable sign may be wet hair where the pet chewed. With light-haired dogs, often the hair is bronzed where they have chewed, especially the hair on their feet, due to pigmented compounds in their saliva.

With rare exception, most atopic pets do not have the typical respiratory signs that people with allergies exhibit, such as runny eyes or noses.

Compounding the problem of atopic dermatitis is the fact that many of these pets have coexisting conditions such as flea allergy dermatitis and skin infections. Allergic skin is more vulnerable to infections. As a matter of fact, pets with chronic skin and ear infections should be checked for atopic dermatitis to see if that is a cause of their chronic infections.

Diagnosis is usually easy; however, some pets with suspected atopic dermatitis may need to have a skin test performed to confirm the diagnosis. This painless procedure involves injecting tiny amounts of various foreign proteins (grasses, pollens, etc.) into the pet's skin and observing any hive reactions that occur. Hives that form at the spots of the injections indicate that the pet is probably allergic to that particular substance. As many as twenty-five or fifty different foreign proteins may be tested at one time; which ones your doctor chooses depends upon the time of year and what part of the country you live in.

Since atopic dermatitis is hereditary, pets with this condition should be spayed or neutered and should never be used for breeding.

In order to determine which allergens your dog may be sensitive to, some doctors perform a blood test in place of the standard skin test. While a blood test can sometimes be a helpful second test in questionable cases, most dermatologists agree that it is an inferior and often inaccurate test when compared with the skin test. Consult with your veterinarian to find out

which test he recommends for your pet.

It should be pointed out that food allergies cannot be diagnosed by skin or blood testing, despite some claims otherwise.

In discussing allergies, it's important for owners to appreciate the summation effect. To simply explain this, let's suppose that your pet has allergies to ten different foreign proteins, such as dust, pollens, and fleas. If eight of these allergens are present at the same time, your puppy will itch and scratch himself. If only seven of these allergens are present, no itching or scratching will occur. This means that if somehow you can avoid several of these proteins, the pet will never itch even though he has allergies. While it's impossible to avoid certain trees in the area when they pollinate, you can minimize exposure to other allergens that might bother the puppy, such as fleas, feather pillows, house dust, and certain houseplants. Since dogs are often allergic to ten or even twenty or more proteins, short of moving to another state, it's impossible for every owner to prevent his pet from coming in contact with many of these allergens.

Treating a pet with allergies depends upon many factors, such as the age of the pet, length of the allergy season (most pets are just allergic during certain times of the year initially, with the allergies often becoming a year-round problem as the dog ages), willingness of the owner to perform the frequent bathing and medicating usually required, and finances of the owner. While the basic treatment is similar for most allergic dogs, every pet is different. Some respond well to the first antihistamine that is tried, while others fail to respond to any antihistamine and ultimately need to be skin tested and placed on desensitization therapy (allergy shots).

Corticosteroids are frequently used as an anti-itching drug for atopic dermatitis. The benefit is that most allergic dogs drastically improve with corticosteroid therapy. There are some bad points to these drugs, however. Short-term side effects, which almost always occur, include excessive eating, drinking, and urinating. Rarely, some dogs will become hyperactive or depressed on these drugs, although most pets show no personality change other than possibly being more energetic (this is because corticosteroids make pets "feel

good"). These short-term effects should not be of enough concern to prevent you from giving them if prescribed. Long-term side effects can include diabetes, osteoporosis, increased infections, Cushing's disease, and Addison's disease (these last two, as well as diabetes, can be serious and even life-threatening). These long-term side effects would only be seen with extremely high doses of corticosteroids, and usually only if the pet had taken them regularly for long periods of time (months to years). Most owners should not shy away from the intermittent use of low-dose corticosteriods when prescribed by the doctor. You should question the doctor, however, if long-acting depot injections are used, or if he fails to mention other, safer forms of therapy for dogs with chronic allergies.

Antihistamines can also be used. Most doctors use these only when other forms of therapy fail to stop the itching or when corticosteroid use becomes excessive. There are many antihistamines, some inexpensive and some fairly costly. Be advised *never* to give your pet over-the-counter medications without instructions from your doctor. This practice can be dangerous or even fatal. A common side effect from antihistamines is drowsiness. It is often necessary for the doctor to prescribe several different antihistamines as well as different dosages and dosing intervals to determine the most effective one. It may be necessary to try five or even ten different antihistamines before finding one that works for your pet.

Fatty acid supplements can also be used. There are several prescription products available from your veterinarian. These products can work well as the only medication needed to control itching in up to 20 percent of dogs. Most dogs need other medications in addition to oral fatty acids to control their allergies. The fatty acids can still help control the inflammation and itching associated with atopic dermatitis by lowering the doses of other potentially more toxic medications. For this reason, even if fatty acids don't help your pet when administered as the only medication, your doctor may still prescribe them as part of the regimen.

Prozyme is an enzyme supplement that increases the digestion and absorption of certain nutrients in the food. Some pets taking Prozyme can get relief from their allergies. As with oral fatty acids, Prozyme is often used as an adjunct to treatment rather than as the sole medication.

While most owners don't relish the thought of frequently bathing their dogs, pets with allergies need frequent shampooing. Remember that many of the foreign proteins that cause your dog to itch are absorbed through his skin. Frequent shampooing decreases his exposure to the problem by removing these sources of itching. Shampooing thus serves as a type of temporary avoidance to the allergens. Most doctors prescribe a regimen of shampooing and conditioning with a medicated anti-itching shampoo and conditioner at least two to three times each week.

Some pets are so allergic that doctors suggest owners not take them outdoors for longer than necessary. Pets that must go outside often benefit from wearing T-shirts and booties to prevent skin contact with grasses and pollens. Washing the pet's feet upon re-entering the house also helps many dogs.

Food Allergy

"Food allergy" has become a catch-all term for many owners and doctors and used whenever a puppy has some sort of medical problem that resolves with a change of diet. True allergy to food is rare. The term food allergy, also called food hypersensitivity, implies that the immune system is reacting to something in the diet. A better term is food sensitivity, which implies an adverse reaction to something in the diet but which does not involve the immune system. Food hypersensitivities can cause reactions involving the skin (most commonly) or gastro-intestinal or respiratory systems. Food allergies account for only about 10 percent of all allergies actually diagnosed in dogs and cats. This 10 percent is the number of cases seen by veterinary dermatologists; most general practitioners feel that food-related dermatitis probably constitutes less than 1 percent of all allergic dermatitis.

While a few dogs with food sensitivities will suffer gastrointestinal disturbances such as vomiting and diarrhea, the most frequent sign is severe itching anywhere on the body, most commonly around the head.

Contrary to what most owners think, pets that are vulnerable to food sensitivities usually develop that sensitivity to a diet they have been eating for a substantial length of time, often well over two years! It would be extremely rare for a pet to develop a true sensitivity to a food that it has been consuming for only a short period of time, although certainly problems, such as vomiting or diarrhea, can develop when a new food is offered, especially if the new diet was introduced suddenly rather than gradually.

When we speak of a food sensitivity or hypersensitivity, we're actually talking about a pet becoming sensitized to certain ingredients in the food, rather than the entire diet itself. Remember that pet food is composed of many ingredients; sensitivities can develop to any of these ingredients. Because proteins are mostly "antigenic," the protein sources in the food are most likely to cause a problem. These protein sources can include any type of meat, including beef, chicken, pork, and yes, even lamb! Other sources that can cause a problem include milk, eggs, wheat, oats, horse meat, cornmeal, and yeasts. In cats, fish and dairy products are most often blamed. Food additives account for only about 5 percent of food sensitivities; this means that buying "additive-free" foods does little to help control food sensitivities. Food processing can make a food more or less likely to cause a reaction in dogs. Because a sensitivity to ingredients in the food often takes a year or more to develop, food sensitivities and hypersensitivities are problems that are not encountered in most puppies.

Owners are often surprised to hear that a pet can develop a food sensitivity to lamb and rice diets, which are touted as hypoallergenic. (For more on lamb and rice diets, see Chapter 5, "Feeding Your Puppy.")

You may want to reconsider before spending extra money on these hypoallergenic diets for a few other reasons as well. Many lamb and rice diets also contain pork, beef, chicken, or egg as well, which are potential allergenic protein sources as well. Finally, consider this: If your pet is eating one of these lamb and rice diets that contains other protein sources, and then develops a food allergy, what will you feed it? A pet that develops a food sensitivity eating a lamb and rice diet doesn't have many food

choices left. Other diets that can be offered should include a protein source the animal has not eaten before, which means you will have to spend a lot of money on diets that contain fish, rabbit, venison, lobster, crab, or shrimp.

Your doctor may suspect a food sensitivity in your itchy dog if it fails to respond to conventional treatments such as corticosteroids or antihistamines. Signs you may notice in your dog include generalized itchiness, redness, especially on the face, feet, and abdomen, itchiness and redness of the ears, and sometimes itchiness just of the facial area. Food sensitivities are diagnosed by the doctor performing a food elimination trial. The doctor will prescribe either a commercial hypoallergenic diet or he may give you a recipe for you to prepare a diet at home in order to aid in the diagnosis. An elimination trial with a hypoallergenic diet is tried only after other diagnostic tests, such as skin scrapings for mange and fungal cultures for ringworm, have been done to eliminate these more common diseases. The diet should be the only thing your dog eats for at least four and in some cases twelve weeks. If the itching resolves while she is eating the special diet, food sensitivity is the likely cause of her problem. Some dogs have a partial resolution of their itching when on a special diet; this indicates that a food ingredient is only partly responsible for the itching, and other tests must be done to determine other causes. Other tests that are used when diagnosing a food sensitivity include skin tests and RAST or ELISA blood tests. These tests are highly inaccurate and should not be used as the sole determinant. With regard to the RAST or ELISA blood tests, a positive result does not have much meaning. A negative test, however, does imply that the offending food protein is unlikely to be causing the problem.

If a food sensitivity is diagnosed, the doctor may suggest slowly adding new ingredients to the hypoallergenic diet to see if the itching resumes. If it does, then your dog is sensitive to that ingredient. This particular ingredient is taken off of the list of things your pet can safely eat. Once all of the sensitive ingredients have been determined, the doctor will work with you to put together a diet your pet can eat without itching.

Since this introduction of various foods takes a lot of time and patience, some doctors will recommend keeping your dog on the hypoallergenic diet used in the feeding trials for the rest of its life.

Parasites

Internal Parasites

Intestinal parasites, commonly called worms, are very common in puppies. It has been suggested by experts at the Centers for Disease Control that 100 percent of puppies are infected with roundworms or hookworms. Since parasites occur commonly in puppies, it's important for owners to have a thorough understanding of the problem.

The most common parasites that occur in puppies are roundworms, hookworms, tapeworms, giardia, and coccidia. Giardia and coccidia are not worms but rather protozoan organisms. Transmission of all parasites involves direct contact with another infected pet. For puppies, the most common source of infection is the mother dog or a littermate.

Roundworms

Roundworms can cause illness and even death in puppies if a sufficient number of worms are present. The worms take nutrients from the puppy's intestine that would otherwise be used by the puppy for growth. Your puppy might acquire roundworms from his mother through her feces, through the placenta prior to birth, when nursing, or from its littermates by ingesting a small amount of their fecal material.

Signs of roundworm infection can include a pot-bellied appearance, rough hair coat, diarrhea (occasionally an adult worm, which resembles a piece of spaghetti, is seen in the diarrhea), coughing (due to the immature worms migrating through the lungs), and vomiting (the vomit often contains one or more worms). Many cases of roundworm infections are diagnosed in normal puppies through a microscopic fecal examination, or "stool" test.

The parasites can also cause health problems in humans, who can ingest the infective eggs in the puppy's feces, stool-contaminated soil, or from contaminated hands or objects. While this sounds disgusting, remember that not everyone washes his hands thoroughly after handling a puppy or disposing of its fecal matter. Most commonly, children who don't have good hygiene and who frequently eat dirt are infected. Several things can happen to an infected child:

- In most cases the infection is asymptomatic, which means there are no signs of illness and the person doesn't even know he is infected.

- Two distinct diseases can be seen after ingestion of roundworm eggs. The first is visceral larval migrans, where the larvae (immature worms) migrate through various body tissues. Signs of the disease depend upon which tissues are affected, but commonly fever, liver enlargement, and increased white blood cells (specifically the eosinophils, which often increase in parasitic disease) and gamma globulins are seen. In ocular larval migrans, the second syndrome, the eye is involved. Since this syndrome closely resembles a certain type of eye tumor which can occur in children, correct diagnosis is even more important.

Roundworms are easily treated in puppies and dogs with

the correct type of anthelmintic, or deworming medication, prescribed by your veterinarian. Owners should avoid using over-the-counter dewormers available at pet stores, as these products may not work. Owners who plan to breed their female dogs should consult their veterinarians regarding a regular, prophylactic deworming schedule for the mother and puppies.

Hookworms

Like roundworms, puppies become infected with hook-worms by eating infective eggs or larvae (found in another pet's stool or vomit), from transfer through the mother's placenta, or through the mother's milk while nursing. Because a single worm can produce 200,000 eggs a day, and most pets can be infected with one to several hundred worms, transmission of this parasite occurs quite easily. Mature dogs (over 6 months old) that might ingest infective eggs or larvae do not develop problems; the eggs or larvae do not develop into adult worms in the intestines but rather encyst in various muscle tissues, as do roundworms. In a female adult dog, pregnancy can activate the cysts, causing the larvae to migrate across the

placenta and into the developing puppy. By the fourth postpartum week, most of the larvae have developed into adult worms in the puppy's intestine and now produce eggs to infect the environment.

Hookworms commonly cause anemia in puppies. In fact, this may be the most common cause of puppy anemia. The disease is most often diagnosed in a routine fecal examination, although it should be highly suspected in any puppy that is lethargic and has pale or white gums.

In humans, hookworms can cause a syndrome similar to the visceral larval migrans condition seen in roundworm infection. Most commonly, hookworms cause a cutaneous larval migrans syndrome. The hookworm larvae enter the skin after direct contact with infected soil (as commonly happens when walking barefoot through the yard, mud, or sand). Typically, a "creeping eruption" pattern develops in the skin, where the larvae are migrating through the skin.

Hookworms are easily treated using drugs similar to those used to treat roundworms. If you plan to breed your female dog, consult your veterinarian regarding a regular, prophylactic deworming schedule for the mother and puppies.

Whipworms

Whipworms, so named because their tail whips around in a dog's large intestine, are rarely a problem in puppies under 1 year of age due to their long and unusual life cycle. Signs of whipworm disease include diarrhea, with or without blood and mucus. Some dogs have vague intestinal signs, such as excessive gas, abdominal cramping ("colic"), or weight loss. Diagnosis involves several microscopic fecal examinations as the eggs are often difficult to detect. Treatment involves an appropriate deworming medication.

Tapeworms

Tapeworms can occur in puppies, but they are much less common than roundworm and hookworm infections. The most common cause of tapeworm infection is ingestion of infected fleas. Fleas often feed on dog feces. If a dog is passing tapeworm segments containing eggs in the feces, the flea becomes infected with tapeworms. Your puppy then eats the flea and becomes infected.

Tapeworms are easy for owners to diagnose but are often difficult for the doctor to detect. Unlike the other worms, eggs are not laid directly in the feces but rather are contained in the tapeworm segments seen in the feces. The segments resemble grains of rice; when first laid, they are white, about 1/2 inch long, and alive. With time, the segments die and resemble brown rice. Owners who detect tapeworm segments in their pet's feces or on the hair surrounding the anus should contact their veterinarian for the appropriate deworming medication. Humans can only be infected with this type of tapeworm by accidentally ingesting a flea!

Coccidia

Coccidia are microscopic, one-celled protozoan organisms. They are a common cause of diarrhea, which is often bloody, in young puppies. They are transmitted by direct contact with infected feces.

Coccidia are easily diagnosed with a microscopic fecal examination. Treatment involves an appropriate medication for ten days. Owners are not in danger of contracting coccidiosis from their puppies.

Giardia

Like coccidia, giardia are microscopic protozoan organisms. Unlike coccidia, they are often difficult to diagnose. As many as three fecal specimens may need to be examined before the organisms are seen. Many older pets probably harbor the giardia organisms in their intestines without ever showing any signs of illness. As is true with many intestinal parasites, disease is more likely to be seen in and be more severe in puppies. Often the disease is treated despite a negative fecal test if it is suspected. This disease can cause diarrhea, bloating, and gas in puppies. The diarrhea often has a "cow-patty" appearance, is pale and very foul-smelling. Weight loss and poor body condition are also symptoms. Humans can get this disease by direct contact with infective feces; campers are frequently infected by drinking water from streams or ponds where animals eliminate. Giardia is treated with oral medication, usually metronidazole, prescribed by your veterinarian. Some cases of giardia are not cured with standard doses of metronidazole. Because of this, and because some pets can show signs of toxicity with higher doses of the drug (including vomiting, diarrhea, unsteady gait, and seizures), fenbendazole is another choice. Most small puppies are treated with furazolidone, which is more palatable and easier to administer than the bitter-tasting metronidazole.

Heartworms

If the truth be known, heartworms should probably be named lung worms or blood vessel worms. That's because in most cases, the worms actually live in the pulmonary (lung) vessels. Worms are only found in the heart in severe infections, where they start out in the blood vessels of the lungs and "back up" into the heart. However, when heartworms were first discovered most dogs probably had such severe infections that many worms were seen in the heart as well as the pulmonary vessels, and the name heartworm was born.

This disease almost never occurs in puppies, due to the long life cycle. However, it's important to know about it because your new puppy will need to take medication to prevent this disease from ever occurring.

Heartworms are transmitted by the bite of a mosquito. When a mosquito bites a dog that has heartworms, it transmits some of the microscopic baby worms (called microfilariae) as it feeds on the dog's blood. These microfilariae go through several molts or growing stages in the mosquito's body. After the molts, the mosquito can transmit the disease to the next dog it bites if that dog is not regularly taking a preventive medication.

After the dog acquires the larval heartworms from the mosquito, the larvae spend about six months slowly making their way to the dog's heart and pulmonary vessels. About six months after the mosquito bite, the dog has adult heartworms living in its pulmonary vessels, heart, or both, depending upon the number of worms present.

Since it takes at least six months from the time of the mosquito bite (assuming the mosquito is carrying the baby heartworms) until the first adult heartworms are seen, a dog would need to be at least 6 months old before it could ever have a heartworm infection.

Heartworm disease is easily diagnosed with a blood test for heartworms, which is done during your dog's yearly visit for checkup and vaccinations. There are two types of heartworm tests: a filter test and an "occult" or adult test.

The filter test checks for the baby heartworms (microfilariae), whereas the occult test checks for adult worms. Which test is run depends upon what type of heartworm preventive medication (daily or monthly) your dog is taking. Pets taking the daily medication need an annual filter test; those taking the monthly medicine need an occult test. Stray dogs over 6 to 8 months of age need both tests run, because occasionally one of the tests can be negative and one can be positive. Since we want to be sure a dog doesn't have heartworm disease, both tests are needed for older pets not currently taking any preventive medication and who have missed several doses of medicine. Testing a dog prior to starting the preventive medicine is important for two reasons. First, if the dog has heartworms, you need to know this before starting preventive medication and developing a false sense of security. Second, some types of preventive medicine can cause an allergic and sometimes fatal reaction in dogs that are positive on the filter test. As a rule, if your dog has heartworms, it needs to be treated before starting preventive medication.

The most common signs of heartworm disease include coughing, lethargy, loss of appetite, and weight loss. But dogs can be diagnosed with heartworms even if they are asymptomatic (not acting sick). In rare cases, a dog can die suddenly, usually during physical activity, such as running or chasing a ball, without showing any signs of the disease.

Treatment, at the time of this writing, involves four intravenous injections of an arsenic-type drug. Prior to treatment, a dog undergoes a battery of laboratory tests, including blood tests, a urinalysis, EKG, and chest radiographs (EKG). These are done to determine if other diseases are present that might complicate treatment. If everything looks OK, your dog will spend several days in the hospital undergoing treatment. While most healthy pets suffer no ill effects from the heartworm treatment, some dogs can get sick and, in rare cases, die. After the treatment, if your dog was diagnosed as having baby heartworms as well as adult heartworms, it will need a second treatment in six weeks to kill the baby worms. During this recovery period at home (the six weeks after the adult treatment while waiting for the baby worm treatment), you must keep your dog as quiet as possible. Any physical exertion can release a lot of the dying adult worms and cause pulmonary embolization, which can be fatal. Pulmonary embolization occurs when a ball of dead heartworms travels to and blocks a pulmonary vessel. Signs of pulmonary embolization include coughing, fever, loss of appetite, and lethargy. After completing the treatment, you should start administering heartworm preventive medication to prevent the disease from recurring. Since adult heartworm treatment doesn't always kill every worm, your dog will need another occult test a few months after treatment. If this test is positive, another round of treatment may be needed, but this is highly individual and depends upon each unique situation. In the future, we hope to have heartworm treatments that are easier to administer and cause fewer side effects than the arsenic drug currently available.

Puppies are placed on preventive medicine on the first puppy visit. Some doctors choose to wait before prescribing heartworm medication until the second or third heartworm visit; however, current recommendations by the American Heartworm Society dictate beginning the drug on the first visit at about 8 weeks of age. Depending upon where you live, your dog may need to take the medicine only a few months of each year, during the so-called "heartworm season." Other pets need to be on the medicine year-round to prevent heartworms.

Pet owners may choose either a daily or monthly form of the medication. Choose whichever form is easiest for you to administer. The monthly form is a bit more forgiving: if you miss giving the daily medicine by even 48 hours, your puppy can contract heartworms. With the monthly dosage, if you miss the dose by a few days your pet is usually still protected. You should discuss the options with your doctor and choose whichever form you are most comfortable administering. The medicine is available in a pill form, which must be given just like other pills, or a chewable tablet form that the puppy will eat just like a treat.

Most owners don't realize that heartworm medication is a prescription drug. You can't buy it at the store, and you can't just walk into any veterinary hospital and ask for it. You must have a valid doctor-client-patient relationship in order to purchase the drug, which means your dog must have been examined and tested for the disease by the doctor within the past year. If you're planning on moving, it would be a good idea to stock up on enough medication to last until your pet's next annual visit.

External Parasites

Mange

Mange is a very common parasite infection of the skin. The parasite is a microscopic insect called a mite. Actually, there are two common types of mange.

The first, demodectic mange, is the most common one in puppies.

Demodectic mange is caused by the *Demodex canis* mite. All puppies acquire these mites from close contact with their mother shortly after birth. In most cases, the mites live quietly in the hair follicles of the skin, never causing any problems. All puppies have demodectic mites in their hair follicles. Only a few will actually develop the disease called demodectic mange.

There are three forms of demodectic mange: a localized form, where only one or two spots of skin are affected, a generalized form, where the entire body is affected, and an adult-onset generalized form, where in adult dogs the entire body is affected. These adult dogs usually have an underlying disease (cancer, liver disease, hypothyroidism, diabetes), or some form of immunosuppression that allows the mites to cause mange.

Puppies develop demodectic mange as a result of a suppressed immune system, which allows the mites that would normally live quietly in the hair follicles to reproduce out of control. The resulting inflammation is seen as mange. The disease is not usually itchy (unlike sarcoptic mange, discussed below), unless a secondary bacterial infection is present (which is sometimes the case).

While many breeds of dogs are prone to developing demodectic mange, it is commonly seen in Shar Peis, bulldogs, Doberman pinschers, Great Danes, and German shepherd dogs.

Initially, the disease causes mild hair loss, sometimes associated with a reddening of the skin. If not diagnosed and treated at this stage, there are two possible outcomes: the disease may stay localized, causing one or a few bald spots that may resolve without treatment; or the spots may spread, causing a generalized form of the disease.

Since demodectic mange closely resembles two other common puppy skin diseases, ringworm and bacterial folliculitis (a bacterial hair infection), a skin scraping is needed to look for the mites. Skin scrapings reveal the mites in most cases of demodectic mange, which allows for a quick, easy, and painless diagnosis; rarely a skin biopsy is needed to confirm the disease.

The localized form is usually treated with a topical prescription medication. The generalized form is currently treated with a special dip that kills the demodectic mites. The dipping is expensive. Most pets require four to eight dips. However, dipping is continued until a skin scraping fails to reveal the mites, and then at least two more dips are done to make sure all the mites have been eradicated. Relapses of demodectic mange can be seen and must be treated early and aggressively. Secondary bacterial infections are treated with oral antibiotics. Affected dogs should not be bred and it is recommended they be spayed or neutered, as this disease is hereditary. This type of mange is not transmissible to other dogs or people.

The other kind of mange is called sarcoptic mange, named after the mite that causes the disease, *Sarcoptes scabeii*. Unlike demodectic mange, which mainly occurs in puppies, sarcoptic mange can occur in any dog regardless of its age. Also unlike demodectic mange, this disease is very itchy, and skin scrapings may fail to find the mite up to 50 percent of the time. This disease, unlike demodectic mange, is also very easily transmitted to other dogs and pet owners by close contact with an infected dog or its bedding.

A skin scraping is diagnostic 50 percent of the time. If the scraping is negative but sarcoptic mange is still suspected, the disease is treated and the puppy's response (or lack of response) to treatment can confirm the presence (or absence) of the disease.

Signs seen with sarcoptic mange include hair loss and crusted areas of skin. These crusted lesions are especially prominent on the ear margins, elbows, ankles, and breastbone. Most of these pets are extremely itchy and often fail to improve significantly with standard anti-itching medication (corticosteroids). Many dogs also have secondary bacterial skin infections that must be treated.

Treatment involves a medicated dip, similar to the regimen for puppies with demodectic mange, or oral or injectable ivermectin drug therapy. Ivermectin can be fatal in collies, shelties, Old English and other sheepdogs, and mixes of these breeds; dipping is used for these pets. Additionally, ivermectin is not approved by the FDA for treating mange; nevertheless, many drugs used in treating pets are not FDA approved but are safe and effective when used properly under veterinary supervision. Unlike demodectic mange, sarcoptic mange usually responds quickly to therapy. However, it is a disease which is easily misdiagnosed, since it resembles other skin diseases, and as many as half of the skin scrapings used to make the diagnosis may not reveal sarcoptic mange mites.

Ear Mites

Ear mites are another form of mange, but most often only the ears are affected. This condition is caused by a mite called *Otodectes cynotis*. The disease is readily transmitted between pets of various species. I have seen several cases in which there was no known exposure to another pet for some time. Rarely, ear mites can be transmitted to owners.

A puppy with ear mites usually will shake its head a lot and scratch its ears. Lifting up the ears for a look usually will reveal a large amount of dry, black, crusty exudate resembling dried dirt. The disease is very itchy and the puppy is quite uncomfortable.

The doctor can easily diagnose the infection by looking in the ear with a special instrument called an otoscope (the same thing your doctor uses to look in your ears). The mites are usually seen during the otoscopic exam.

An ear swab needs to be examined microscopically as well, for two reasons. First, occasionally the mites are not seen with the otoscope but they or

their eggs are seen microscopically after swabbing the ear. Second, ear mites often cause secondary bacterial or yeast infections that should be treated as well as the mite infection.

Treatment involves a thorough medicated ear flushing to remove the crusty debris. Medicated ear drops can be used; a newer treatment involves using oral or injectable medication, which can be used in conjunction with the drops. Because mites can live outside of the ear canals temporarily, pets treated with ear drops should also be treated with a flea spray to kill the mites. Ear drops should be given for at least one month which is twice as long as the treatment for other ear diseases; flea spray may also be needed during the course of treatment to kill any mites living outside the ears on the puppy's body. The most common reasons for a pet not to recover from ear mite infections are:

1. Incorrect diagnosis. Treating the ear for mites when in fact the problem could be a bacterial or fungal infection. Microscopic examination of the ear swab will quickly show the difference.

2. Incorrect treatment. Treating the ears for less than one

month with the correct ear drops will often result in failure to cure the problem.

Fleas

Depending upon where you live, fleas may or may not be a big problem. If your puppy has fleas, proper flea control is essential. Avoid advice from friends and pet store employees who are not properly trained in flea control. Fleas are a medical problem and as such require a consultation with your doctor, a medical professional who has been trained in parasitology, pharmacology, and toxicology. Every pet owner's situation is different; and there are no flea programs that work on every pet in every situation. Consulting with your veterinarian to develop a flea control specific to your own unique situation makes sense. Not only that, but he or she probably has a few products that are not available in pet stores. The following information will arm you with the basic facts you need to know about flea control; consult with your doctor for a flea control program customized to your pet's needs.

Prior to starting flea control, thoroughly steam clean your house or apartment at the beginning of the flea season and at the end of the season. This will remove the flea eggs that regular vacuuming won't remove.

1. Begin flea control by vacuuming and mopping the house or apartment.

2. Then, treat *all* pets by bathing and dipping with products recommended by your veterinarian. Bathing and dipping is done every two weeks; alternatively, using ProSpot plus a Program flea pill is preferred for dogs and can actually *prevent* fleas when used at the start of the flea season! The flea pill, which prevents flea eggs from hatching, is given monthly at the same time you give your puppy its monthly heartworm pill. Use ProSpot every two weeks and *do not dip your dog!*

3. Treat the inside of your house or apartment and the outside (yard) *at the same time* you treat the pets. Your veterinarian may recommend sprays, foggers, borate-based powders (to provide year round flea control), a professional exterminator, or some combination of these methods. A new product, Interrupt flea spray, is a non-toxic, chemical-free yard spray that is very safe and effective for killing fleas. Since 95 percent of the fleas are off of the pet and in

the environment, treating the environment is the most important part of the treatment.

4. Use an approved flea spray (applied with a Brushette for maximum effectiveness and minimum waste) or a flea foam on your pet as directed.

5. Flea collars are ineffective by themselves unless used in conjunction with a comprehensive flea program. Electronic collars are also ineffective, as are garlic and brewer's yeast.

6. Repeat as directed by the doctor.

ABOUT FLEA PRODUCTS: Many flea products purchased at stores are ineffective, used incorrectly, or more toxic than products available through your veterinarian. Pet owners who use store-bought products that fail to kill fleas actually end up spending more money than those who start out with the correct products recommended by their veterinarian.

Controlling fleas is not easy or cheap but by following this information, you should be able to keep your pet relatively free of those irritating little pests.

Fungal Diseases
· ·

Ringworm

Ringworm is one of the three most common puppy skin diseases (the other two are bacterial folliculitis and demodectic mange). It is not caused by a worm but rather by any of several types of fungi. Ringworm is most commonly caused by transfer of the fungus between pets. However, certain types of ringworm live in the soil and pets (and people) can acquire it through contact with the soil.

Ringworm is so named because the classic skin lesion is a circular, or ring, lesion. It is hairless and often has crusting at the center of the ring and almost always at the periphery of the lesion. Like demodectic mange, ringworm can occur as just one or a few lesions or can spread and involve the entire body.

Diagnosis is made by culturing affected hairs and some of the scales from the lesion. The culture normally is positive within five to seven days if ringworm is the cause of the disease; some cultures may take two to four weeks for the fungus to grow. If ringworm is suspected, the doctor may begin treatment prior to culture confirmation. As with demodectic mange, there are several options for treatment. For a few small lesions, often topical treatment with an antifungal medication will work. The generalized form needs more aggressive therapy, including antifungal shampoos and oral medication (which can be expensive). Long-haired animals often need to be thoroughly clipped prior to starting treatment to ensure the best chance of success. The puppy is treated until it appears "cured" (which may take one or more months of aggressive and expensive treatment), and then for at least two more weeks or until another culture fails to grow ringworm.

Ringworm can be carried asymptomatically (the pet has the ringworm fungus on its body but doesn't show signs of disease), especially by kittens. The ringworm fungus is constantly present in our environment, yet only a few puppies ever show signs of the disease. A suppressed immune system or exposure to a large dose of fungus is often the cause for illness. While ringworm is often passed from pet to owner, too many pets are blamed for causing ringworm in children, when in fact another child is often the culprit. A pet suspected of causing ringworm in a person should always be examined and cultured for the fungus prior to starting expensive treatment.

Miscellaneous Diseases

Intestinal Obstructions

Because puppies are by nature curious, and because like human infants they are prone to chewing on various objects, intestinal obstructions by foreign bodies are more common in puppyhood than at any other time in your dog's life. Any number of objects can be attractive to your puppy and end up in its stomach or intestinal tract. These include play toys, pieces of play toys, small balls, metal objects, jewelry, and string. Rubber and plastic objects are commonly swallowed. These obstructions can be prevented by keeping certain objects, such as jewelry, out of harm's way, and by making sure the size of the toy fits the dog (i.e., not offering a 40-pound retriever puppy a toy manufac-tured for a 5-pound poodle). Owners should check their puppy's toys as they would a

---

FIRST AID AND EMERGENCY KIT . . . .

It's often convenient to have a small first-aid kit available for minor problems. You can make one yourself and store the supplies in a fishing tackle box, or buy one already assembled at the drugstore.

In all honesty, in a true emergency there is very little any pet owner can do at home other than stop major bleeding, assist in breathing, and get the puppy to the doctor as soon as possible. For minor problems, the following information can assist you.

Bleeding   Stop the bleeding. For cut nails, use styptic powder or liquid, corn starch or flour, or bar soap. Never trim nails unless you have some type of styptic. Make sure your doctor shows you the proper way to trim nails. In general, if the bleeding doesn't stop within ten minutes, see your veterinarian.

For more serious bleeding from cuts, direct pressure on the bleeding area for five to ten minutes should stop the bleeding. Large gashes may require suturing and should be seen to by the veterinarian. You can bandage minor wounds, although bandaging is more difficult with dogs than people because of their anatomy and the fact that many puppies will chew the bandages. If you apply a bandage, especially on a limb, make sure it's not too tight or the blood supply can be interrupted.

Not Breathing   If your puppy isn't breathing, prompt veterinary attention is needed. You can blow into the nostrils while holding the mouth closed (once every five to ten seconds). Try to feel for a heartbeat over the chest just behind the elbows near the breastbone. If no beat is felt, you can try CPR by laying the puppy on its side, laying one hand on the underside of the chest and one hand on the upper side of the chest where the heart is located, and pressing your hands together at least one compression per second. (You might ask your veterinarian to demonstrate this technique.)

child's to make sure pieces of them (bells, eyes, etc.) are not easily removed. Stuffed animals should not be used as a toy.

Signs of intestinal obstructions are often vague. Vomiting, especially continued vomiting of a projectile or a nonproductive nature, can indicate an obstruction. In general, the puppy often doesn't show signs other than vomiting until the condition has persisted for 24 hours or more. This is dangerous; obstructions lasting for several days often cause perforations or rupture of the intestines, which can lead to peritonitis and rapid death. In some puppies, abdominal pain or tenderness can be detected. The veterinarian may even be able to feel the obstruction.

Diagnosis usually requires radiographs (X-rays); in some instances, a barium swallow may be needed to detect rubber toys or partial obstructions. In rare cases, an abdominal exploratory surgery is needed to confirm the suspected obstruction.

Most puppies survive an intestinal obstruction if it is diagnosed early and treated aggressively. Obviously, this is a condition that is better prevented.

POISON CONTROL ....

Hopefully you will never need to consult with your doctor about poisoning in your puppy. However, because a puppy is curious and often gets into everything, it may become accidentally poisoned. As with children, prevention is the best cure: don't administer over-the-counter medications without your veterinarian's advice and keep all potential poisons locked up.

If you suspect that your puppy has been poisoned, the best thing you can do is call your veterinarian (or the emergency clinic if after hours) as poisonings are usually true emergencies.

You can also call the National Animal Poison Control Center at 1-800-548-2423 or 1-900-680-0000; both calls cost about $30 and can be used by veterinarians or pet owners. Make sure you keep these numbers, as well as the numbers of your veterinarian and the nearest animal emergency clinic, easily accessible.

Anal Sac Disease

Puppies have two anal sacs located at their anal opening. If you imagine the anus as a clock face, the sacs would be located at approximately the 4 and 8 o'clock positions. These sacs are hidden within tissue that surrounds the anus.

Many people mistakenly refer to the anal sacs as anal glands. Dogs do have *anal glands*; however, these are separate and distinct from the anal sacs which often cause problems.

Each anal sac contains glands which produce a foul-smelling liquid secretion. This liquid is stored in the sacs until a bowel movement occurs, at which time the sacs are emptied of their glandular secretion. The function of these anal sac glands is to impart a characteristic odor to the feces, which aids in marking a pet's territory.

Problems arise when the sacs fail to empty. It is not always known why the sacs sometimes fail to empty properly, but the problem seems to occur more in small breed dogs than large breed dogs. When the sacs don't empty properly, they fill up with the glandular secretions and cause the pet discomfort. Clinical signs seen at this point include the pet scooting its rear end on the ground (in a futile attempt to empty its sacs) or excessive biting and chewing at the rear end (both of these signs can also be seen with tapeworm infections).

If you take your dog to the doctor at this stage, he can simply evacuate the sacs during a digital rectal examination. If signs are not seen or are ignored at this stage, the sacs can become impacted and even infected and abscessed. Abscessed anal sacs result when an opening forms in the sacs through the skin; blood and pus ooze from this abscessed area. Treatment for impacted or abscessed sacs is a bit more involved. Often sedation is needed to clean the impacted or abscessed sac. Oral and topical antibiotics are needed to treat the condition as well.

Some pets need to have their anal sacs emptied regularly by the veterinarian. How often your pet will need this done can only be determined by how frequently the sacs fill up. While groomers often say that they empty the sacs during the grooming visit, they usually evacuate the sacs manually from the outside skin surface of the pet. While this can help sometimes, most pets need the internal cleaning of the sacs that only your veterinarian can perform.

Hot Spots

Acute moist dermatitis, commonly referred to as "hot spots," is a common problem in dogs and occasionally in puppies. The condition occurs when some irritant causes the puppy to itch or bite itself excessively. Within hours, a moist, fiery red lesion is seen on the puppy. A common cause of hot spots is flea infestation; hot spots are also seen in long-haired dogs that become hot and itchy, usually in the warm and humid summer environment. Hot spots can also be seen after grooming and are often referred to as razor or clipper burns. What usually happens is that the puppy's hair was clipped close to the skin; the puppy has probably lived with a longer coat for some time, and this shorter coat causes the puppy to itch. Owners can prevent this by having their puppies groomed at regular intervals (every 4-8 weeks) and asking the groomer not to do a close clipping, especially of the face.

Regardless of the cause (which isn't always determined), hot spots should be treated soon after discovery. These lesions are extremely uncomfortable for the puppy; if not treated soon after discovery, they can easily enlarge and become infected.

Most of the time the veterinarian will clip the area and clean it with a medicated solution. An injection of a corticosteroid is usually given to decrease the itching. Medication that is sent home may include a short round of oral corticosteroids to control further itching and a topical product to give the puppy some relief. Many veterinarians use antibiotics on the bigger hot spots, as these are often infected from bacteria introduced by the puppy's excessive licking. In rare cases, the puppy may need tranquilization or an Elizabethan collar for a few days to discourage chewing the lesion.

Chapter 11

Congenital Medical Problems

· ·

Congenital conditions are, by definition, any medical problems that are present at birth. They may or may not be hereditary. Even though they may be present at birth, they may not be detected by the owner or veterinarian until the puppy is a bit older (a classic example of this is a heart defect).

Congenital problems occur fairly rarely in dogs. Some may be insignificant and not require medical correction, such as small umbilical hernias. Others can be life threatening, such as heart conditions. Most congenital conditions require a diagnosis by a veterinarian; this once again emphasizes the need for frequent veterinary visits and complete physical examinations during the first few months of your puppy's life.

Musculoskeletal Conditions
· ·

Hip Dysplasia

Hip dysplasia is probably the most common musculoskeletal problem in large breed dogs. Hip dysplasia, or hip dislocation, is an abnormality of the hip joint. The hip joint is a ball and socket joint: the head (ball) of the femur (large thigh bone) fits into the acetabulum (socket) of the hip, forming a joint. An abnormality of the ball, socket, or both can allow the ball to slip out of the socket, making walking difficult and painful. As the degree of "slippage" (dislocation or dysplasia) progresses, arthritis occurs as new pieces of bone are formed around this joint in an unsuccessful attempt to prevent further "slippage."

While hip dysplasia can occur in any dog, it is most commonly seen in fast growing, large breed puppies, usually puppies whose adult body weight is over 30 pounds.

The cause is multifactorial, which means that many factors, including genetics, nutrition, and environment, can cause the condition. If you plan to purchase a purebred large breed puppy from a breeder, make sure you get OFA certification for the parents of the puppy.

The OFA, or Orthopedic Foundation of America, is a foundation that registers dogs based on skeletal conformation. Any owner of a large breed dog who wishes to breed that dog should have it registered with the OFA. Registration occurs after the owner's veterinarian evaluates the dog under anesthesia. The veterinarian will radiograph (X-ray) the hips and perform orthopedic manipulations of the joint, trying to dislocate it manually. The radiographs are sent to the OFA, where board-certified radiologists examine the hip joints. The hip joints are given a grade after the radiographs are reviewed by several OFA radiologists. This grade then is registered with the OFA. Breeders should furnish the OFA grade to prospective puppy buyers. Of course, if the adult dog receives a poor or failing OFA grade, that dog should not be used for breeding as its puppies stand a chance of having hip dysplasia.

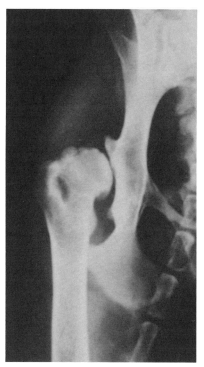

X-ray showing severe hip dysplasia

A disadvantage of buying your puppy from a pet store is that there is no way to know the OFA grade of the parents. However, reputable pet stores will guarantee that their puppies are free from hip dysplasia for up to two years of age; at that time, you should take you dog to its veterinarian for hip dysplasia evaluation. Even if the veterinary evaluation, hip radiographs, and manipulation are normal, your dog could still develop hip dysplasia, as no test is perfect. However, if veterinary evaluation reveals normal hips, the chance of your dog ever developing hip dysplasia is rare.

Assuming the parents of your puppy have normal hips, you could still *cause* dysplasia in your puppy. Remember that hip dysplasia is not only genetic but environmental as well. If you push your puppy to grow rapidly by overfeeding it, you may cause dysplasia. Likewise, if you exercise your puppy strenuously every day, you may cause dysplasia. Hip dysplasia results when the bony growth of the hip joint exceeds the growth of the surrounding muscles which help hold the ball in the socket. Extremely rapid growth may result in excess skeletal growth

at the expense of muscle growth, causing unnecessary pressure and strain on the hip joints, which might lead to hip dysplasia. Frequent discussions with your veterinarian about proper diet and exercise can help prevent this problem.

There are several treatments for hip dysplasia. Conservative treatment involves strict confinement and rest, and analgesics for hip pain. Mild cases of hip dysplasia may improve with conservative treatment, although most veterinarians favor surgical correction for young, growing puppies.

There are several surgeries. Which one might be recommended for your pet depends upon several factors, including your financial situation and the preference and experience of the surgeon. The surgeries either attempt to make the hip joint normal or remove the ball part of the ball and socket mechanism to prevent further pain and arthritis.

A relatively new surgery is called the TPO, or triple pelvic osteotomy. In this procedure, the pelvis is cut and rotated, allowing more socket to cover the ball part of the joint. This surgery is only performed on young dogs, most often between 6 and 18 months of age. It is for this reason that veterinarians recommend hip evaluation and radiographs between 6 and 18 months of age. If the tests are negative at this age and you still want to breed your dog, the hips should be evaluated again at 2 years of age and registered with the OFA.

Signs of hip dysplasia depend upon the severity of the problem. Many puppies walk normally but have abnormal hips when evaluated radiographically or with orthopedic manipulations of the hips. Most of these puppies do very well following TPO surgery. Other puppies with more severe signs have trouble walking, running, getting up and down, and/or turning around. Most of them also do well following surgery.

Even if you decide against surgery for your dog, he should still be evaluated between 6 and 18 months of age. This is because if your puppy has hip dysplasia and you do nothing for it now, you will have to make a decision at some point in its life regarding treatment. The problem will not go away on its own and will get worse. Many older dogs that have asymptomatic hip dysplasia as puppies become arthritic as they age. Pets with severe pain from the dysplasia

can develop a bad temperament and become aggressive. At this point, surgery (but not TPO surgery) is still an option. Medical therapy using anti-inflammatory drugs and a diet to reduce obesity if present may also help. Some dogs unfortunately must be euthanized due to the severity of the problem and pain associated with the arthritis. While it's obviously best to prevent problems with early diagnosis and treatment, hip dysplasia that is not treated in puppies will cause problems with age. As an owner, you need to be aware of this and prepared for it.

Osteochondritis Dessicans

Osteochondritis dessicans, or OCD, is another common musculoskeletal problem of large breed, rapidly growing puppies. OCD is a degenerative condition that can affect many joints, although the shoulder joints are most commonly affected. OCD is caused by defective cartilage maturation. As the puppy grows, bone is formed from pre-existing cartilage. If some of that cartilage is injured, it may fail to properly form new bone. This retained cartilage on the exposed joint surface is what causes the problem.

The shoulder joint consists of the head of the humerus (the upper bone of the arm, also called the funny bone) and the depression of the scapula, or shoulder blade. If retained cartilage is present on the head of the humerus, it can become traumatized as the head of the humerus slides on the depression of the scapula during movement of the shoulder (walking and running). Repeated trauma and pressure to this cartilage area causes pain and difficulty walking and running. Occasionally the cartilage can partially break off, forming a flap in the joint cavity, which can lead to further inflammation and pain.

Diagnosis requires veterinary evaluation. As with hip dysplasia, the shoulder joint is manipulated, not in an attempt to dislocate it as with hip dysplasia, but rather to check for pain when it is manipulated. The shoulder is also radiographed to check for the cartilage lesion that causes the problems. Because both shoulders can have the problem even though only one leg is lame, both shoulders are usually evaluated. Occasionally a radiograph is inconclusive. In this case a special radiograph using

dye may be needed, or the shoulder may need to be explored surgically based on suspicion of the disease.

Treatment is surgical. During surgery, the doctor will remove any diseased cartilage and cartilage flaps. Most puppies recover completely following the procedure. Surgery should be performed soon after diagnosis to prevent secondary arthritic changes from occurring.

Patellar Luxation

Patellar luxation is the term applied to a dislocation of the knee cap (patella). This condition most often occurs as a congenital condition in small breeds of puppies, including miniature poodles, Yorkshire terriers, toy poodles, Chihuahuas, Pomeranians, Pekingese, and Boston terriers. With patellar luxation, the kneecap dislocates over the shin bone (tibia). The dislocation can be mild and not cause any clinical signs, or can be so severe as to cause the leg to "lock" in a fixed position where the puppy has to carry it in the air.

For mild cases not showing clinical signs, your doctor may or may not recommend surgical correction. In severe cases, surgery is needed to correct the cause of the dislocation. Since there might be several different abnormalities that allow the patella to luxate (dislocate), there are several types of surgeries that can be used to correct the problem; often several abnormalities that caused the dislocation are corrected during the same surgery. Your doctor can discuss the specifics of the surgery he may recommend.

Elbow Dysplasia

Elbow problems usually occur in large breed puppies, similar to the hip problems also seen in these breeds. As with hip dysplasia, elbow dysplasia is an inheritable disease. Affected puppies should be spayed or neutered and not used for breeding. You should have your puppy checked and OFA certified for this when his hips are checked. There are two problems commonly associated with elbow dysplasia: a fragmented coronoid process (FCP) and an ununited anconeal process (UAP).

The coronoid process is a small projection of bone located on the ulna, one of the two bones in the forearm. The anconeal process is a projection of bone located on the ulna, the bone in the forearm which articulates with the humerus (bone of the upper arm, the "funny bone"). This process, through its articulation with the humerus, allows movement at the elbow joint.

During bone development in puppies, these processes start out as cartilage that unites with the larger bone (radius or ulna) and becomes ossified (calcified) into bone. During this transformation from cartilage to bone, the process may fail to unite or may become separated from the larger bone due to repeated trauma, as is often seen with excessive exercise.

Puppies with either FCP or UAP exhibit lameness, pain, and sometimes swelling of the elbow. German shepherd dogs, Saint Bernards, and basset hounds are commonly afflicted with ununited anconeal process; Newfoundlands, golden retrievers, German shepherd dogs, and Saint Bernards are most commonly afflicted with fragmented coronoid process.

Treatment involves surgery to either remove the fragmented process or sometimes reattach it to the bone.

Eye Conditions

• •

Cherry Eye

Cherry eye, the slang term for Harderian gland prolapse, often occurs in small breed dogs, especially cocker spaniels, English bulldogs, basset hounds, beagles, Shih Tzus, poodles, and Maltese breeds. The prolapse, or protrusion, most commonly occurs between 3 and 12 months of age.

The Harderian gland is located on the underside of the dog's third eyelid (which functions as a protective barrier against eye trauma). Sometimes the gland will flip over and appear as a red swelling in the corner of the eye nearest the nose. Because it resembles a cherry, it was named cherry eye. The condition may be inherited.

While the condition is not serious, it should be treated. Very rarely, eye drops can make a tiny cherry eye improve. Usually, surgery is needed to correct the condition. Surgery can involve removal of the gland or suturing it to the eyeball. Removal of the gland may predispose the eye to a condition called keratitis sicca, or dry eye, as this Harderian gland does make some of the tears that coat the eyeball. However, dry eye most often occurs in dogs with both Harderian glands. Consult with your veterinarian regarding which procedure he feels is best for your puppy.

Entropion/Ectropion

Entropion is a condition where one or both eyelids roll inward toward the eye. The lower outer edge of the lid is most frequently affected. The chow chow, bloodhound, Labrador retriever, English bulldog, Doberman pinscher, Chesapeake Bay retriever, Saint Bernard, Rottweiler, poodle, Irish setter, and Shar Pei breeds are predisposed to congenital entropion.

In ectropion, one or both lids roll outward away from the eye. Ectropion usually involves the lower eyelids. It is common in the bloodhound, Saint Bernard, American cocker spaniel, basset hound, and bulldog.

Both conditions result from excess laxity (looseness) of the skin and musculature of the lids.

Mild ectropion may not require surgical treatment. Entropion is more serious. Since the eyelids are covered with hair, an inward rolling of these lids places the hair in direct contact with the eyeball, causing ulcers and scratches of the eyeball. Surgery is needed to correct both entropion and severe cases of ectropion. To prevent "overcorrection" of entropion, it is usually advised to delay surgery if possible until the puppy is 4 to 6 months old; often, mild cases will correct themselves as the puppies grow. If the eye is ulcerated from contact with the eyelid hair, it is treated as well.

Tear Staining

Some small breeds of dogs, especially poodles and Maltese, normally have excess tearing. You may notice that the face on either side of the nostrils is wet and the hair, especially white hair, is discolored a brown or copper color. This often occurs in small breed dogs with poor eyelid closure during blinking and an abnormal lacrimal "lake" in the eyelids. Since the tears don't drain properly, they flow onto the facial skin. Usually no treatment is prescribed other than regular cleaning of the tears and face; although surgical correction may be attempted in more severe cases.

Occasionally there is an abnormality of the nasolacrimal ducts, the ducts that normally drain tears from the eyes into the nostrils. Sometimes this occurs when the tear ducts are infected or inflamed, causing them to become clogged with mucus. Occasionally, the tear duct is not normal and can't function properly; surgery may be needed to correct the abnormality or make a new hole for the duct to drain the tears.

CERF

CERF stands for Canine Eye Registry Foundation. As with the OFA, the CERF registers dogs that are prone to inheritable eye conditions, such as collies and Shetland sheepdogs (for "collie eye anomaly," a disease of the retina very common in these two breeds) and retrievers (which are prone to "progressive retinal atrophy"). Puppies of these breeds, especially those intended for breeding, should be given a thorough eye examination. Other inheritable eye diseases such as glaucoma and cataracts (common in beagles, poodles, and cocker spaniels), may also occur in your puppy if any of his ancestors had these conditions.

Heart Conditions
• •

Congenital heart problems occasionally occur in puppies. These heart problems are most commonly diagnosed during the physical examination when the doctor auscults, or listens, to the heart and lungs with a stethoscope. Normal heart sounds are described as a "lub-dub;" occasionally, the doctor may hear a heart murmur which sounds like a swooshing sound ("lub-swoosh," "swoosh-lub," or "swoosh-swoosh"). A heart murmur is caused by abnormal, turbulent blood flow through the heart or vessels leading from the heart. Blood flow can become turbulent under several conditions:

1. A blood vessel is narrowed;

2. A hole is present in the wall of the heart;

3. Heart valves are leaky, allowing blood to flow backward—out of the heart—instead of forward—through the heart and into the vessels leading to the lungs (pulmonary artery) or body (aorta).

Sometimes, the doctor may hear an "innocent" murmur. This is a soft murmur that usually disappears by 4 to 6 months of age and is not a sign of heart disease.

Depending upon the loudness (intensity) and location of the murmur, the doctor will usually have some idea what type of congenital heart problem exists.

Patent Ductus Arteriosus

A patent ductus arteriosus, or PDA, occurs when the ductus arteriosus remains patent, or open. This is the most common congenital heart problem in puppies. The ductus, a short fibrous tube, normally is open in the fetal puppy while it is inside its mother's uterus. It diverts blood that would normally go to the lungs and be oxygenated to the aorta and general circulation (puppies get their oxygen from the mother, so their lungs don't need to work until after they are born). Shortly after birth, the ductus should close on its own. If it fails to close (remains patent), blood flow will be shunted from the aorta into the pulmonary artery and lungs, resulting in excess blood flow to the lungs and subsequently the left side of the heart.

The condition is most common in female puppies and is hereditary in poodles, German shepherds, Shetland sheepdogs (Shelties), collies, Pomeranians, and spaniels. Without treatment, heart failure will occur, and 50 percent of affected puppies will die by 1 year of age.

Treatment is surgical and involves tying the ductus closed. If surgically corrected shortly after diagnosis, the prognosis is excellent, although the procedure is somewhat risky. Sometimes the ductus is thin-walled; while attempting to tie it, it can rupture and the puppy can bleed to death. Even with this slight risk, the surgery is necessary to correct the problem.

Aortic/Pulmonic Stenosis

The aorta is the blood vessel leading from the left side of the heart that supplies blood to the rest of the body. The pulmonary artery is the vessel leading from the right side of the heart, taking blood to the lungs where it is oxygenated and then returned to the left side of the heart by way of the pulmonary veins. Sometimes a part of either the aorta or pulmonary artery is stenotic or narrowed. When this occurs, blood is under increased pressure trying to leave the heart. The heart must then exert extra pressure to force the blood through the narrowed opening in the artery. Heart failure can eventually result. Aortic stenosis is hereditary and most commonly occurs in Newfoundlands, German shepherds, boxers, golden retrievers, and German shorthair pointers. Pulmonic stenosis occurs in many breeds, particularly beagles, bulldogs, Chihuahuas, and fox terriers.

Treatment depends upon the severity of the problem. Puppies with a mild narrowing and not showing clinical signs can often lead a normal life without any treatment. Dogs with moderate to severe narrowing are more likely to show signs and require surgical correction. Several surgical procedures are available; all attempt to increase blood flow through the narrowed artery. With surgery, most puppies will live full, healthy lives.

Ventricular Septal Defect

A ventricular septal defect is the medical term for a hole in the heart. The hole occurs in the muscular tissue (ventricular septum) that separates the left and right ventricles. Small holes cause no problems. Larger defects are associated with a significant shunting of blood from the left side of the heart to the right side. This results in increased blood flow to the lungs and subsequently the left side of the heart. As with other heart defects, heart failure eventually results without treatment. While this is the most common congenital heart defect in kittens, it is fairly rare in puppies.

For larger defects, surgery is needed. Open heart surgery is one option, although cost prohibits most owners from choosing this option and a special surgical center is needed for the procedure as it involves heart bypass techniques. Another procedure that is less technically demanding is called pulmonary artery banding. Good results occur with this technique.

Persistent Right Aortic Arch (PRAA)

Persistent right aortic arch occurs when the right fourth aortic arch, which normally degenerates after birth, persists in the puppy. This arch causes problems by encircling and trapping the esophagus. Since the esophagus is narrowed, food doesn't pass into the stomach normally and regurgitation occurs. This is similar to megaesophagus. There is evidence of a hereditary basis for this condition, as it occurs in German shepherds and is also common in golden retrievers.

The condition is diagnosed with a barium swallow radiograph. Treatment involves surgery to cut the aortic arch. Prognosis is generally good if surgical correction is done early.

Miscellaneous Congenital Conditions

Umbilical Hernia

A hernia is a hole in the body wall; an umbilical hernia is a hole in the umbilical (belly button) area. Umbilical hernias are most often congenital; while the hole is present at birth, the herniation (material sticking through the hole) may not develop until later in life. Some breeds are predisposed to umbilical hernias, including Airedale terriers, basenjis, Pekingese, pointers, and Weimaraners. Since umbilical hernias can be hereditary, affected dogs should not be bred.

Most puppies with umbilical hernias have small hernias with only a small amount of abdominal fat sticking through the hole. Very small hernias usually cause no problems and don't have to be corrected, although they often are when the pet is spayed or neutered. Larger hernias should always be corrected. If not corrected surgically, there is a chance other tissues such as intestines could become entrapped in the hernia. Also, any trauma the puppy might experience later in life (such as a fall or if accidentally struck by a car) could enlarge the hernia even more, causing serious problems.

Cryptorchidism/ Monorchidism

By birth, the testicles of most male puppies have descended into the scrotum. Occasionally, this happens shortly after birth or within a few weeks of birth. Sometimes, something goes wrong and one or both testicles fail to descend into the scrotum. If both testicles fail to descend, the condition is called cryptorchidism and the puppy is a cryptorchid. Far more common is the condition in which one testicle descends but the other does not; in this situation, called monorchidism, the puppy is a monorchid.

Testicles need to be located in the scrotum or the retained testicle is infertile. However, retained testicles still produce the male hormone testosterone beginning at puberty. Retained testicles have a much higher incidence of cancer than scrotal testicles; all animals with one or both testicles that are retained need to be neutered. The hidden testicle is often located in the abdomen, but occasionally it is located just underneath the skin in front of the scrotum (the inguinal or groin area). Since the retained testicle can be located anywhere in the abdominal cavity, the surgery to remove it combines a normal neutering for the scrotal testicle and exploratory surgery to remove the retained one. Monorchid dogs should not be used for breeding as they can pass this condition on to their male offspring; it is also considered unethical to breed monorchid dogs. Cryptorchid dogs, being infertile, cannot father offspring.

Megaesophagus

Megaesophagus means "enlarged esophagus." The esophagus is the tube which carries food from the mouth into the stomach. This is a congenital problem in puppies and is usually first seen as regurgitation when the puppy begins to switch from a liquid diet to solid puppy food at weaning, usually at 4 to 6 weeks of age. The condition is a defect in the neuromuscular functioning capability of the part of the esophagus located near the stomach. It is hereditary in certain breeds such as wire-haired fox terriers, miniature schnauzers, and German shepherd dogs. The regurgitation usually occurs immediately after or even during feeding, although in rare cases the puppy may not regurgitate for several hours after feeding.

Diagnosis is with a barium swallow radiograph (X-ray). Megaesophagus must be differentiated from a condition causing similar signs, persistent right aortic arch, PRAA. (See page 130, Heart Conditions).

The only treatment available is medical care of the puppy; surgery is ineffective. Feeding small amounts of food, trying various types of diets (soft, liquid food or a hard diet), feeding from an elevated position, and giving certain medications to speed passage through the esophagus and stomach can all be tried. Many puppies do not respond well to this treatment and are often euthanized.

Chapter 12
Lifeplan

• •

One of the most important things veterinarians can do for their clients is inform them what medical care their pet will need throughout its life and the associated costs. While this book focuses on puppies, this chapter is about adult dogs as well as puppies. In the next few pages you will find a description of the care your puppy will need as it grows into adulthood, mid-life, and its golden years as a geriatric pet. By knowing what care your puppy will need throughout its life, you can better plan ahead.

2 Months Old (8 Weeks)

First veterinary visit (although this can also occur at 6 weeks if you acquire the puppy then):

• Complete physical examination

• First puppy vaccinations: distemper-hepatitis-leptospirosis-parainfluenza-parvo virus-corona virus (DHLPP-C)

• Fecal exam for intestinal parasites

• Heartworm medication administered

Heartworm medication is started on the puppy's first visit, depending upon the area of the country you live in. Heartworms are easily prevented with a daily or monthly chewable medication. In some areas of the country, the medicine is administered during "heartworm season," which is generally the warmer months of spring and summer. In other areas, "heartworm season" is year-round and the medication must be administered on a yearly basis for the life of the dog.

3 Months Old (12 Weeks)
Second veterinary visit:
• Complete physical examination
• Second puppy vaccinations: DHLPP-C, kennel cough, bordetella
• Heartworm medication administered

4 Months Old (16 Weeks)
Third veterinary visit:
• Complete physical examination
• Third puppy vaccinations: DHLPP-C, kennel cough, rabies
• Fecal exam for intestinal parasites
• Heartworm medication administered
• Six- to eight-month supply of heartworm medication prescribed

The estimated cost for the first three puppy visits is approximately $180.

4-6 Months Old
• Spaying or neutering
• Tattooing

Tattooing serves as a permanent form of identification in the event that the pet is lost or stolen (some estimates are that one in four dogs will become "lost" at some point in their lives). Tattooing is painless and is most often performed when the puppy is spayed or neutered. The tattoo, an identification number, is usually placed on the inside of either hind leg. If your puppy will be a show dog, check with his breed registry to determine if there are any requirements regarding where he can be tattooed. More important than the tattoo is the registry; make sure the tattoo is registered with a national pet tattoo registry. Some doctors prefer "microchipping," the insertion of a tiny chip under your puppy's skin, instead of tattooing; consult your doctor.

The estimated cost for the spaying or neutering and tattooing will vary with the size of the pet at the time of surgery. The cost is approximately $135.

6-18 Months Old
• Orthopedic evaluation for hip and elbow dysplasia in puppies 30 pounds and larger.

Puppies that will weigh over 30 pounds as adult dogs are prone to hip dysplasia. Early evaluation through radiography (X-rays) and orthopedic manipulation can often detect any problems before your puppy shows clinical signs of limping or arthritis. Early surgical intervention can be performed when hip or elbow dysplasia is detected between 6 and 18 months of age.

The cost for the orthopedic evaluation is approximately $90 which includes the necessary anesthesia, radiographs, and orthopedic manipulations.

12 Months Old

At 12 months of age, your puppy is now an adult dog. This is true for most puppies; some of the larger breeds, such as Great Danes and retrievers, actually continue to grow until about 18 months of age. For these larger breeds, what applies at the 12-month visit would still apply, except that the diet would remain puppy food until about 18 months of age.

At 12 months of age, your puppy will go for its one-year visit, often called a birthday exam. During the visit, the doctor will perform a thorough examination of your now adult dog. Your veterinarian will discuss important health and wellness information with you at this visit such as the following:

• • ➡ The puppy should be switched to an adult maintenance diet. Adult dogs do better if fed two or three small meals each day, especially large breed dogs (over 40 pounds) that can easily develop bloat, a fatal condition of the stomach. Smaller breeds can have food available all day, as long as they are used to this type of feeding and do not become obese. Obese pets will be started on a medically controlled diet.

• • ➡ Heartworm medication should be given year-round for the life of your dog. This is especially true along the Gulf Coast; depending upon where you live, your doctor's recommendations may differ.

• • ➡ Continue daily vitamins. Many doctors start puppies on Prozyme, an enzyme supplement, to aid in digestion and absorption of nutrients; decrease food intake by 10 to 20 percent after one month if your dog gains weight. Continue the Prozyme for the life of your pet to maximize nutrient absorption from its diet. Prozyme may also help your pet's coat look better and decrease excess shedding.

• • ➡ Start your pet on ProSpot and the Program flea pill in April to prevent flea problems in the summer. All dogs, especially indoor pets which are more likely to develop severe reactions to fleas (flea allergy), need to take ProSpot until October; the

Program flea pill is given monthly for the life of your dog. (Flea season in Texas runs April through October. Consult your own veterinarian for specific information on parasite control in your location.)

••➡ Dogs weighing 30 pounds or more need to be checked for elbow and hip dysplasia if this has not already been done. This is usually done between 6 and 12 months of age. After a short-acting anesthetic is given, the hips and elbows are manipulated and radiographed (X-rayed) to check for dysplasia. A positive finding indicates the need for corrective surgery.

••➡ The next set of vaccinations, fecal check, physical examination, and heartworm test occurs in four months (at 16 months of age) and annually thereafter. The baseline blood profile will also be done at this time. The purpose of this blood profile is to find out what is normal for your pet. While normal values are established and published in veterinary books, your pet may have a value outside the normal range yet not have any diseases. Establishing what is normal for your pet will help when your pet gets sick and a blood profile, done at the time of illness, can be compared with the normal, baseline profile.

••➡ Dogs that have not been spayed or neutered need that done now. Early (4-6 months of age) spaying and neutering can

TRAVELING IN THE CAR . . . .

It is important that your puppy travel well in the car. While most owners don't take their pets everywhere with them, they need to be comfortable enough so that the trip to the veterinarian is pleasant.

Start by taking your puppy on frequent short trips in the car. Getting your puppy used to short trips at an early age will prevent future "car sickness" and will make traveling easier. To prevent the fear of traveling that many pets have, be sure to take them in the car to places other than just the doctor's office, such as the park. If the puppy associates the car with a fun, pleasant experience at an early age, it shouldn't have any trouble riding in the car when it is older.

prevent medical problems (such as breast cancer in female dogs and prostatic disease and testicular cancer in males) and behavioral problems. Most pets have been spayed or neutered by 1 year of age. Some owners may put it off thinking they want to breed their pets but then change their minds. No matter how old your pet is, it's never to late to have the surgery done!

••➡ If you plan to breed your dog, the ideal time is usually between 2 and 5 years of age (especially for females). A follow-up hip and elbow evaluation and registry with the Orthopedic Foundation of America (OFA) is necessary for large breed dogs at 2 years of age.

••➡ The first oral surgery for dental disease is performed at age 2-3, and annually thereafter. Dental disease is the most common disease in dogs; early diagnosis, treatment, and home care are critical to saving your pet's teeth, gums, and jaws, and preventing the spread of harmful oral bacteria throughout the body.

••➡ At 8 years of age, dogs are considered "mid-life" pets. They need a mini-blood profile and often a urinalysis at least every

---

FEAR OF FLYING. . . . .

Occasionally an owner wants to take a puppy on the plane for a trip. Each airline has its own requirements and should be contacted at least one month prior to traveling. Following are a few general tips that can make the trip go smoother for you and your puppy:

1. Most airlines require a health certificate from the veterinarian stating the puppy is healthy enough to fly. Generally, the certificate should be obtained within 10 days of the trip.

2. Many pets do better when sedated. Your doctor can discuss sedation with you. Because no two pets require the same dose of medicine nor act the same when on the drug, you might consider a trial dose a few days before the trip to make sure you get the desired effect (mild sedation).

3. Puppies can usually travel in a carrier under your seat if the carrier fits comfortably there. Otherwise, they travel in the cargo hull of the plane, which is pressurized for comfort.

one to two years until 12 years of age. The results of this blood test will be compared to the initial baseline profile done when the pet was vaccinated at 16 months of age. Any changes may indicate early kidney or liver disease, diabetes, or cancer.

•• ➡ At 12 years of age, dogs need a complete blood profile annually. As costs allow, they should also get a urinalysis, EKG, and chest radiographs (X-rays) annually to look for signs of kidney, liver, and heart disease, and cancer, which are more common in older pets. Early diagnosis prevents pain and suffering and is less expensive than treatment of an ill or dying pet.

This lifeplan is advised for all dogs, although your own veterinarian's recommendations may differ slightly. Regular veteri-

nary visits and laboratory testing are needed to prevent serious disease. As with humans, preventing disease is preferred to treating a disease; it is also much less expensive.

The annual cost of veterinary care obviously will differ depending upon the needs of your own specific pet. For example, while most pets need their first oral surgery (ultrasonic dental scaling) for periodontal disease at 2-3 years of age, some dogs build up tartar (infection) much slower. They may not need the surgery until 4-5 years of age. Their care would be less expensive than that of a pet that requires annual ultrasonic scalings starting at 2 years of age.

As an approximate estimate, for the typical 30-pound dog that requires two veterinary visits a year (one for its annual vaccina-

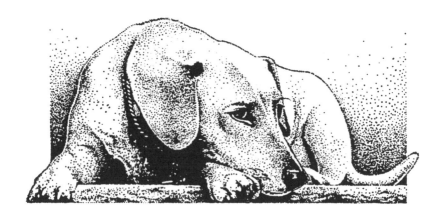

tions and examination, one visit for a minor illness), a dental ultrasonic scaling each year, and a 12-month supply of heartworm medication, the approximate cost would be $300. This does not include major illnesses, food, grooming, boarding, toys, or treats. While $300 may seem like a lot, realize that you do not normally spend this on one visit but rather over the course of a year. Also keep in mind that this amounts to less than $1 per day, which is not much to spend on the pet you love.

Recent surveys indicate the average dog owner is willing to spend approximately $550 per year on his pet.

When It's Time to Say Goodbye

At some point in your pet's life, you may be faced with the difficult decision to euthanize your dog. Usually, the pet is older and has been ill for some time. In some cases, a puppy must be euthanized for medical or financial reasons.

Most veterinarians do not like the term "putting the pet to sleep." The pet is not going to sleep; it is being killed, its life is ending. Young children who hear the term "put to sleep" may be shocked when the pet doesn't wake up. Some are terrified that when they go to sleep they will end up like the pet and not wake up. Be honest with your children. While euthanasia is difficult for all involved, it is an opportune time to explain death and dying to young children and help them come to accept this natural part of living.

The process of euthanasia, while a painful decision for owners, is a simple one. Most of the time the process involves a painless intravenous injection of an overdose of an anesthetic agent. The pet quickly and quietly becomes unconscious; breathing ceases, and the heart stops beating within a minute or two.

Owners often inquire about being present during the procedure. Most doctors are not opposed to this, but you should carefully consider whether this is truly what you want. Many owners don't want to see their pet dead and would rather remember the good times they had with their pet. For others, being present when the pet dies is comforting to them and their pet and helps them with the grieving process. If you choose to be present, here are a few things to remember:

• The procedure is painless; the only thing your pet feels is the needle being introduced into the vein, similar to when it gets a shot or has blood drawn.

• Pets pick up on your emotions. While it may be hard to contain your emotions during the procedure, the pet will be more comfortable if you can postpone grieving until the procedure is completed and the pet is dead.

• Rarely, some pets may make sounds during the procedure, exhibit muscle twitching after the procedure, or eliminate feces or urine. These are rare occurrences but can be discomforting to owners. Rest assured that if these events occur, they occur *after* death; the pet is totally unaware of them, has no voluntary control of these functions, and feels no pain.

After euthanasia, the pet's body must be disposed of. Several options are available:

• Some owners choose to take the pet home and bury it in the yard. While many cities have laws prohibiting this, it is unlikely your doctor would turn you in for choosing this option. If you choose home burial, remember to bury the pet several feet underground in a container so that other animals or pets cannot dig up the body.

• The other option, more commonly selected, involves the hospital disposing of the pet. This may be done through the city's animal control office or a pet cemetery, which cremates the body and disposes of the ashes. Owners can also choose a more elaborate option such as private cremation, where the ashes are returned to you in an urn for private burial in a grave.

Chapter 13

Lowering the Cost of Pet Care

● ●

Everyone, including doctors, agrees that the cost of medical care is high. Even medical care for our furry friends can be expensive at times. While every owner would like to get the best care for his pet at the lowest price, going to the "lowest bidder" for pet health care can be a mistake!

As an owner, you and you alone will have to decide whether low cost or high quality is more important. If you choose higher-quality care, there are still things you can do to lower the cost of health care and not sacrifice quality or service. Keep in mind that the average cost of health care for a 30-pound dog (excluding major illnesses) is about $300 per year. While

studies show that the average pet owner is willing to spend approximately $550 per year on a pet, the following suggestions will help you cut that cost without sacrificing quality of care.

1. Have your dog examined and vaccinated at least annually. Annual examinations and vaccinations are the least expensive way to prevent diseases that can easily cause severe illness and in some cases kill your pet. A dog can be fully protected against the major communicable diseases for under $100 a year. And where should you take your pet for these vaccinations? As a rule, it's no more expensive (and in some cases it's less expensive) to go to a full-service animal hospital than a low-cost vaccination clinic.

2. All dogs should receive heartworm preventative medication. The cost for heartworm treatment is about $500; for a fraction of that cost you can prevent this deadly disease.

3. Practice preventive medicine. Common sense tells us it's cheaper to prevent something than fix it. Disease prevention costs little compared to the cost of treating a sick pet. Periodontal disease is the most common disease in pets. Regular dental cleanings will prevent more serious problems (abscesses, sinus infections, etc.). Since the incidence of expensive and serious diseases increases as our pets age, annual geriatric examinations and blood and urine tests for our older pets are needed to allow early disease detection.

4. Get pet health insurance. No pet should be euthanized because an owner can't afford medical care. Pet health insurance is extremely inexpensive and allows owners the opportunity to have expensive procedures such as cancer chemotherapy performed when the alternative might be death for the pet.

5. Open a savings account for your pet. You don't want to pay for health insurance? Open a bank account for your pet instead. At $1 per day, funding this account for just five years will create a nest egg for "pet emergencies" of $1,825 (not including interest). If you think this idea sounds silly, consider this: the money in the account is more than most owners will ever need to spend for emergency care for their pets. When your pet dies at the ripe old age of 15-20 years old, close the account and spend the balance on yourself! If nothing else you are saving money for something; if your pet doesn't need it you have a nice little nest egg to enjoy.

6. Ask your doctor about ways to cut health care costs. Many doctors offer money-saving programs while not cutting the quality of care. For example, some doctors offer referral incentive programs. For each new client you refer, both your friend and you save 10 percent on your next visits. This can allow you to save a little on every visit; the more new friends you refer, the more you save!

Other doctors offer multi-pet discounts: if you own two or more pets and have them vaccinated at the same time, your bill is discounted based on the number of pets.

Another cost-cutting idea we developed for our clients is a VIP, or Very Important Pet, program. Each time you visit, your total bill is recorded on a VIP card. When you fill up your card, you receive credit on your next visit for the average amount you spent on prior visits. This allows you substantial savings, yet you receive excellent medical care.

Some doctors offer monthly specials. For example, since February is Pet Dental Health Month, some hospitals offer a reduced price on teeth cleanings during that month. This allows you to save a little money on a much-needed service.

Saving money is important to everyone. Veterinary medicine can offer advanced diagnostic tests and treatments for many serious diseases; however, these can be expensive. Cutting costs of health care can be done without compromising care. Considering the suggestions in this chapter will allow you to offer your pet high-quality care at an affordable price.

Chapter 14

Common Puppy Breeds

. . . .

If you decide to purchase a pure-bred dog, there are many breeds (over 150) from which to choose. This chapter is a discussion of the attributes of some of the most popular breeds I treat in my busy practice. If your breed isn't listed, I encourage you to visit with your veterinarian and check out the American Kennel Club (AKC) book of dog breeds at your local library. Learn everything you can about the breed of puppy you wish to purchase before making your buying decision. One word of warning: pure breeds usually have more medical problems than mixed breeds. Don't be scared by the number of possible problems listed in this chapter. Any pet can become ill, and there is never a guarantee that just because a certain breed has specific problems common

to that breed that your new puppy will necessarily develop similar problems.

COCKER SPANIEL

This popular breed of dog comes in two varieties: the American cocker and the English cocker. The American cocker is the most popular in our country; the English cocker has a longer face than its American counterpart and is usually a slightly bigger dog. Common coat colors include shades of silver, black, buff, red, chocolate, and tan.

Once America's most popular breed, cocker spaniels developed medical and behavioral problems (poor disposition, aggressiveness, many hereditary problems) as a result of inbreeding. Now many of these problems have been resolved and the cocker spaniel is once again becoming a friendly, popular breed. When selecting a puppy, it is important to try and observe the parent dogs. Disposition is important in these dogs; avoid any puppies whose parents are standoffish or aggressive.

Common Problems
Aggressiveness, submissive urination, dental malocclusion, cataracts, autoimmune hemolytic anemia, glaucoma, miscellaneous eye problems involving the lids (entropion, ectropion, cherry eye) or tear production (keratoconjunctivitis sicca, commonly called "dry eye"), luxating patellas (dislocating kneecaps), hip dysplasia (usually affecting the larger cockers), atopy (skin allergies), seborrhea, ear infections, hypothyroidism, intervertebral disc disease.

CHINESE SHAR PEI

These unusual looking dogs were popular several years ago. They became the "cool" or "in" breed. Many of these puppies sold for several thousand dollars. The Chinese Shar Pei dates back to the Han dynasty; the excessively wrinkled skin was developed as protection when fighting. The breed became nearly extinct in China as it was used for food and its skin used for coats. Shar Peis are noted for chronic skin and eye problems; many are aggressive as well. Predominant coat colors are black, cream, fawn, and red.

Common Problems
Aggression, skin diseases due to excessive skin folds (demodectic mange, staphylococcal infections, seborrhea, hypothyroidism, skin allergies (atopy), mucinosis, eye problems (keratoconjunctivitis sicca, commonly called "dry eye"), eyelid problems including entropion, respiratory problems due to narrowed nasal passages, ear infections, patellar luxations (dislocated kneecaps).

CHOW CHOW

The chow chow, often just called the chow, is an ancient guard dog of China. Distrust of strangers and aggressiveness are common in this breed. Chows have poor peripheral vision and should be approached cautiously from the sides or back. The coat is light at birth and darkens with maturity; red, cinnamon, and black are common coat colors. The tongue is characteristically blue-black; dogs with splotches of blue or black in their otherwise pink tongues may have some degree of chow in their pedigree.

Common Problems

Aggression, hypothyroidism, growth deficiency and sex hormone deficiency, hair loss and hyperpigmentation, eyelid problems including entropion, respiratory problems due to narrowed nasal passages, ear infections, patellar luxations (dislocated kneecaps), hip dysplasia.

COLLIE

Once popular because of the *Lassie* television series, collies originated in Scotland. Collies come in a rough (most popular), smooth, or bearded version. Collies are sweet, enjoyable dogs that love people, especially children. Collies thrive on and need human companionship. Common colors are sable, tri-color, and blue merle. Gray-coated collies are rare and are the result of a defective gene responsible for immune system problems (low white blood cell counts) that eventually result in death.

Common Problems

Small eyes (microphthalmia), "collie eye disease" that may be mild and cause no clinical signs or severe enough to cause some

visual impairment, demodectic mange, nasal solar dermatitis, discoid lupus erythematosis, and dermatomyositis.

RETRIEVER

Labrador and golden retrievers are popular large breed dogs. Both breeds are excellent swimmers, good hunting companions, excellent with families and children, and originated in Newfoundland. Colors for Labradors include black, chocolate, and yellow. Golden retrievers are dark or light golden in color.

Common Problems

Atopic dermatitis (skin allergies), ear infections, hip dysplasia, elbow dysplasia, osteochondrosis, cataracts, retinal atrophy muscular dystrophy and myopathy (Labradors), and hypothyroidism.

LHASA APSO

Lhasas originated in Tibet and were used as guard dogs. Lhasas are often described as aloof and wary of strangers. They can be aggressive, especially around small children. Owners should establish dominance over Lhasa puppies to prevent future aggressive problems.

Common Problems

Patellar luxation (dislocated kneecaps), uroliths (bladder stones), atopy (skin allergies), and lissencephaly (brain damage).

SHIH TZU

The Shih Tzu was a common gift to monarchs in ancient China. Shih Tzus can be nippy if owners do not properly train them as puppies and establish dominance over them. Otherwise, they can be sweet dogs and love to be pampered.

Common Problems

Uroliths (bladder stones), eye problems including cherry eye, corneal ulcers, and lid problems such as entropion.

POODLE

Poodles come as standard, miniature, toy, and teacup varieties. They originated in Europe and come from the German *pudel*

(meaning "to splash in the water"). The smaller varieties were developed from the standard poodle. All poodles are highly intelligent dogs that are popular circus performers. The standard poodle is a fun-loving dog with the typical large-breed dog personality. The smaller varieties are good pets but can become spoiled by pampering owners. All poodles require regular grooming to attain the desired type of cut. Unlike most breeds of dogs, shedding is not a problem with poodles; people with allergies to dogs often choose poodles as pets for this reason.

Common Problems

Hip dysplasia (standard poodle), patellar luxation (smaller varieties), eye problems including cataracts and glaucoma, eyelid problems including eyelash problems and entropion, heart problems (patent ductus arteriosis), and uroliths (bladder stones, smaller varieties).

Index